There's a Flying Squirrel in My Coffee

There's a Flying Squirrel in My Coffee

Overcoming Cancer with the Help of My Pet

Bill Goss
Lt. Commander, USN (Ret)

ATRIA BOOKS
New York London Toronto Sydney Singapore

The author of this book is not a physician, and the ideas, procedures, and suggestions in this book are not intended as a substitute for the medical advice of a trained health professional. All matters regarding your health require medical supervision. Consult your physician before adopting the suggestions in this book as well as about any condition that may require diagnosis or medical attention. In addition, the statements made by the author regarding certain products and services represent the views of the author alone, and do not constitute a recommendation or endorsement of any product or service by the publisher. The author and publisher disclaim any liability arising directly or indirectly from the use of this book, or of any productions mentioned herein.

ATRIA BOOKS

1230 Avenue of the Americas
New York, NY 10020

© 2002 by Bill Goss

ISBN: 0-7434-3729-2

First Atria Books hardcover printing July 2002

10   9   8   7   6   5   4   3   2   1

ATRIA BOOKS is a trademark of Simon & Schuster, Inc.

For information regarding special discounts for bulk purchases,
please contact Simon & Schuster Special Sales at 1-800-456-6798
or business@simonandschuster.com

Unless otherwise noted, all photos belong to the
author's private collection.

Designed by Jaime Putorti

Printed in the U.S.A.

*T*his book is dedicated to my mother, Barbara, my father, Gene, and my aunt, Ann Clark, for inspiring me in so many ways.

To my mother, for her Irish wit, her uncanny ability to make friends with anyone, her tireless efforts raising six rambunctious children on a tight budget, and her love of worldwide travel.

To my father, for his remarkable athleticism and strength, his unsung WW II heroics on Navy ships in the Pacific theater, and his love of deep reading and creative writing.

To my aunt, for her sense of humor, her belief in the power of the human spirit to overcome adversity, and her love of all living things, both great and small.

This book is also dedicated to the firefighters, police officers, rescue workers, military personnel, and civilians from all over the world who gave up their lives due to the terrorist attack on America on September 11, 2001, or its aftermath.

There's a
Flying Squirrel
in My Coffee

1

Going Supersonic

*W*hat if you just finished the most exciting day of your life—a thirty-year dream exploding into a spectacularly exciting reality—then the next day you found out you were going to die? How would you feel? What would you do?

Here's my story.

Being a pilot and breaking the sound barrier was all I ever wanted to do. Now I was going to do it. Now I was about to turn my dream—and the many struggles that followed—into a glorious, exhilarating victory.

Chuck Yeager's historic flight had filled my overactive imagination with an explosion of sound and fury and speed ever since I had first read about it when I was eight years old. I used to tremble with excitement and smile to myself at just the thought of going faster than the speed of sound.

At eighteen, while whipping around the sharp corners and steep hills of Millburn-Short Hills, New Jersey, holding my nose with one hand and holding on for dear life to the back of a garbage truck with the other, the dream of going supersonic still lived vividly within my imagination. I knew no one would have thought a garbage man could fulfill a dream as wildly ambitious as mine, so I kept it to myself.

Many things happened over the next two decades that could have defused my dream, but thankfully they didn't. I enlisted in the Navy and then completed college. A few years later I began flying military aircraft until I had finally progressed to that special place and time in the universe where incredible dreams really do come true.

Now, twenty years after slinging my last trash can, I was going to do it. I remembered for a moment the familiar smell of decay that fanned from the back of the garbage truck, as I now picked up the musky scent of sweat on the ejection seat I was preflighting before takeoff. It was the sweat of the pilot and all the other pilots who had climbed into that Navy F-18 fighter jet cockpit before me.

As I strapped myself into the rear cockpit of the F-18 Hornet, I smiled as I suddenly realized that now I'd be blessing this cockpit, and its future pilots, with *my* scent—sweat exuding from my every pore as I anticipated going higher and faster than I'd ever gone before.

The hundred different things on the cockpit preflight and prestart checklists are good to go. The enlisted man standing thirty feet in front of me gives me and the Marine Corps fighter pilot in the front cockpit the hand signals: It's time to start our engines. But we don't just start jet engines. We ignite them. The engines whine and whir as they begin to spool up, then burst into two 900-degree flames of green-blue-orange-red that are almost indescribable.

Now I'm sitting on top of two colossal torches and all is well with the world. One small fuel-leak rupture and I'd explode into a million pieces like a giant Roman candle. But that thought never crosses my mind, even though I've already survived a major plane crash.

The only thing that crosses my mind is my insatiable need for speed.

The engines start to sizzle. The after-start checklists are completed and we taxi out to the end of a monstrous twelve-thousand-foot runway at a naval air station in Jacksonville, Florida. It's not far from where Peggy and I live with our twins, Brian and Christie, down by the St. Johns River.

I was qualified to fly one of the fastest turboprop airplanes in the world, the P-3 Orion, a spy plane designed to track and destroy ballistic-missile submarines with either torpedoes or nuclear depth bombs, but I still hadn't had—and wouldn't ever get—a chance to break Mach one, also known as the speed of sound, unless I got a chance to fly an aircraft specifically designed to accomplish such a remarkable aerodynamic feat.

I needed an entirely different kind of aircraft for that. The other three types of jets I had the opportunity to fly—the T-2 Buckeye, the TA-4 Skyhawk, and the Coast Guard Falcon jet—couldn't get the job done either.

The job, of course, was to go faster than sound itself. That's 741 mph at sea level, but it all depends on your altitude, the air temperature and air density. We're talking fast. And before Chuck Yeager, we're talking impossible.

Currently the Navy has only two jets designed to go *that* fast. First, there's the older and super-quick F-14 Tomcat, designed to intercept inbound Russian bombers before they can reach the aircraft carrier.

And then there's the newer and extremely maneuverable

F-18 Hornet, a fighter-bomber. It's the jet flown by the Blue Angels, the Navy's crack flight demonstration team, in air shows all over the country. That's the jet I'm strapped into right now. And she's a beauty. Painted camouflage whitish gray to match the cloud cover so that it is almost impossible for enemy fighters to spot her against a slate-colored sky, the swept-wing Hornet costs around $50 million per copy, loaded with the latest computer displays and radar screens that have replaced the familiar cockpit instruments you find in conventional aircraft.

The other guy I'm flying with is a tall, lean, steely-eyed Marine Corps fighter pilot. A friend of mine, Bill Hilgartner, he's known for some time that I've been lusting to go faster than a .45-caliber bullet. This morning we'll be together on a training flight with another jet for the purpose of practicing high-speed tactical flight maneuvering. We'll be conducting this training hop in a large block of airspace reserved specifically for military use over the Atlantic Ocean, off the coasts of southern Georgia and northern Florida.

After taxiing onto the runway and being cleared for takeoff, we ram the dual throttles forward into afterburner. Instantly, red-hot flames blast out thirty feet from the rear of the jet, plastering me so hard into the back of my ejection seat that I couldn't pull myself forward even if I wanted. My eyeballs are forced back into my skull by an indescribable form of induced gravity. That's g force for you.

One-one thousand. Two-one thousand. The fifty-thousand-pound titanium steed rockets down and then leaps off the runway. The pointed nose of the Hornet is angled to the heavens and I watch the ground below disappear at an almost alarming rate as the jet continues to accelerate faster and faster, just like my racing heart, reaching a breathtaking speed in an instant.

The Navy control tower clears our jet out of its airspace and then passes us over to Departure Control. They follow us on radar, helping us to avoid crashing into other airborne craft. Departure Control stays with us until we reach a safe distance from civilization and all those earth-dwelling creatures below.

We then report on our radio that we are "feet wet," meaning that we have just crossed the beach line heading east, out toward the immensity of the wind-swept Atlantic Ocean. In the earliest days of aviation, if I had been flying low and slow enough, I really could have stuck my legs down and gotten my feet wet. But not on this rocket!

In just minutes we are miles off the coast of the Florida–Georgia border, entering special-use airspace reserved for us, an area where we can do maneuvers and fly at speeds that we aren't allowed to do over land. This is because of the serious damage sonic booms cause to people and structures beneath the flight paths of supersonic jets traveling just above the ground. And because the jets are moving faster than sound, there is no advance warning that you are about to be rocked by a sonic boom. It is simply impossible to hear a jet traveling at supersonic speed when it is coming toward you. The jet is moving ahead of and faster than its own sound. You might see it coming, but you will never *hear* it coming. You will definitely hear it leaving.

Sonic blasts are so powerful that they feel like a huge bomb is exploding just over your head. Sonic booms have caused entire populations of turkey farms to drop dead from fear-induced heart attacks. And while we are talking turkey— thousands of turkey lawsuits can be very costly to the federal government. And that wouldn't be good for anybody.

A few minutes later, we are going through some extraordinarily violent flight maneuvers with the two other jets that have joined up with us. A dogfight begins. We blast up to thirty thousand feet and then drop the nose straight down to pursue the other two jets. They're now simulating the bad guys, known in Navy pilot lingo as "bogeys."

I see a tiny speck on the deep blue ocean below. In a second the tiny speck visually explodes in my windscreen into a large fishing boat just as I observe my jet's Mach meter—the speedometer—read .80, then .90, then suddenly *ka-boooom!* as I blast through the sound barrier and rock the poor fishermen in the boat below, giving them—and me—the thrill of a lifetime. I continue to focus on the meter as it passes Mach 1.0, then 1.1.

Enormous beads of sweat pour out from under my helmet as we execute a 6-g pull on the flight control stick to gain back our altitude—effectively changing my body weight from 190 pounds to almost 1,200 pounds in just a fraction of a second. It is so painful that I almost pass out. Yet, for some strange reason, I'm in love with this feeling.

Just a few minutes later we head back for a couple of simulated aircraft-carrier landings at the naval air station. Practice carrier approaches and landings, even on the long runway at the naval air station, are a lot different from the smooth approach, flared landing, and long rollout of a conventional landing. A good Hornet touchdown feels like a crash landing to anyone else. To stay safe, it is important for carrier pilots to continually practice the relatively slow, nose-high approach to the landing zone and the teeth-rattling touchdown required to qualify as a safe landing on an aircraft carrier. The jet's nose-high attitude also dramatically improves the chances that the long metal tail hook hanging from the back of the jet will hook on to one of the four thick steel arresting cables stretched across the flight deck.

If you miss all the arresting cables and don't immediately add max power at the moment of touchdown, your jet will continue rolling down the angled flight deck and off the other end, allowing you and your jet to fall into the deep blue sea. You and your jet will then almost certainly be run over by the gigantic 100,000-ton aircraft carrier, which is sometimes steaming forward at speeds greater than 30 mph during flight operations to create its own wind.

Thankfully, we didn't have to worry about that today, since our runway was surrounded by tall grasses instead of waves. But I have done carrier landings in the open ocean in two other jets, the T-2 Buckeye and the TA-4 Skyhawk, and it is a *huge* adrenaline rush.

After our final landing back at the naval air station, I feel so exhilarated that I laugh hysterically into my oxygen mask at the top of my lungs. From takeoff to landing, the total flight was less than forty-five minutes. We taxi back to the parking area and shut down the engines, then pose in front of the Navy fighter jet for a photograph.

I'm on top of the world. Finally, after all these years, I've experienced the ultimate wild ride of a lifetime—blasting through the sound barrier at the controls of an incredibly sophisticated and tremendously powerful flying machine. For a brief moment I touched the face of God. Nothing gets any better than this. I figured this would keep me on cloud nine for a long, long time.

I figured wrong.

Earlier that month, something the size of a pea had popped up on the back of my left ear and had started to itch. Finally, it bothered me enough to visit the flight surgeon to get it removed.

I remember her telling me not to worry about it. "It's a

harmless fatty cyst," she said. It will be reabsorbed into your body in no time at all."

As I got up to leave, I suddenly felt a strong bolt of premonition. I immediately returned to her office and insisted she remove the bump from the back of my ear.

"Doc, if you don't cut this thing off, I'll do it myself, tonight, using the bathroom mirror and a straight razor."

I remember her looking at me, checking to see whether there was a seriousness or a smile in my eyes. Apparently she saw both.

"Okay, I'll cut it off. But really . . . it's nothing."

In just a few minutes she removed the little nothing from the back of my left ear, which was covered by perfectly unblemished skin that contained some hard white tissue inside. I laughed and joked with her as she put in a single stitch to stop the bleeding, then I was on my way.

That all happened earlier last week and I'd pretty much forgotten about it by now. I mean really, it was only a harmless fatty cyst.

And what about now? Well, I've just gone supersonic. I'm sitting on top of the world. I'm the luckiest man alive.

A few hours later I'm back in my office, working for the admiral, listening to a peculiar recorded message from the flight surgeon. Her normally upbeat and cheery tone has been replaced by a steady, measured cadence. The hair on the back of my neck rises as I sense danger.

"Lieutenant Commander Goss, you have an immediate appointment with Dr. Fischer in the Navy Hospital's Ear, Nose and Throat Clinic."

As soon as possible, I meet with Dr. Fischer. From the look in his eyes, I can tell I am about to be dealt the worst hand I've ever been forced to play.

I notice the sweet-pungent smell of sweat—but this is different from the macho musk in the cockpit. This is the odor of people anticipating doom. This is the smell of fear. The problem is, I can't tell whether it is coming from myself or from Dr. Fischer.

The doctor clears his throat, then tells me the three most dreaded words in the English language:

"You have cancer." . . . *You have cancer.*

Suddenly I feel like I've been dead asleep for centuries, only to be blasted awake in an instant to find myself treading water, alone, in the dark, in the vastness of the Pacific Ocean. I don't know when the sharks and barracudas are going to pull me under and shred me to ribbons, but I know there is no possibility of escape. A feeling of complete and total despair. Over the entire course of my thirty-eight years on earth, which has included many close calls, I have never felt so alone before.

"You could be dead in six months."

Dr. Fischer's words pierce the almost nonexistent air, and I take another empty gulp for oxygen. When he won't return my direct gaze, I suddenly realize that he doesn't believe I *could* be dead in six months. He believes I *will* be dead in six months.

I struggle for some words—any words—to string into a question, just to break the gut-wrenching silence, but nothing comes.

My throat feels very dry. I would love a glass of water, though I know my thirst is unquenchable. This is a thirst for life, and there's no drink that can help.

Dr. Fischer is just as uncomfortable with the situation. He's a healthy-looking naval officer, a lieutenant commander, with a beautiful wife and two young children—just like me. Perhaps he's looking at his own mortality when he looks into my eyes and it's just too difficult for him to face this brutally awful situation head-on.

Finally, under my breath, I mutter, "Well, at least he said six months, not three," as I struggle to maintain a sense of perspective—and a sense of humor. But at the same time I feel myself falling from the top of the world—falling from the heavens in a death spiral, only this time without a copilot to help me pull out just in the nick of time.

Never could I have imagined that at this same moment, a creature the size of a cotton ball was also falling to earth.

And that this tiniest of angels would help save my life.

2

Prognosis Negative

I sat in silence in my car in the hospital parking lot, wondering how I was going to make the drive home to Peggy and our twins. I had so much to tell her and yet I still had so few answers to my own questions. A bombshell had just been dropped into the center of our lives. How would I minimize the collateral damage? I was still thinking like a Navy pilot, rather than like a randomly unlucky guy just given a death sentence. Finally, I turned the key in our old Honda's ignition and began the twenty-minute drive to our house on Fleming Island. Then I began to reflect on Dr. Fischer's words.

He believed I had a very rare form of deadly skin cancer caused by the sun: amelanotic malignant melanoma. I had a melanoma tumor that was without any pigmentation, very unlike the black mole that normally characterizes the disease. Melanoma actually means "black tumor" in Latin.

The likelihood that I had cancer had initially been discovered by Dr. Elie, a pathologist who worked in the basement—The Dungeon—of the large naval hospital I used for my annual flight physical. Dr. Elie had come across a piece of white tissue in a small bottle of formalin that had been sent to him for review a few days earlier. It was labeled "probable sebaceous cyst removed from patient's left ear." Dr. Elie took a tiny piece of the white tissue out of the little biopsy bottle, squashed it between two small glass slides, and slipped it under his microscope. What his highly trained eyes saw was something that was definitely *not* sebaceous-cyst-related cells. He stained the cells and again looked at them under his microscope. This time he saw something he recognized not only as the unusual cell-growth patterns related to cancer but specifically to skin cancer, and even more specifically to malignant melanoma. He then wrote in his pathology report on the hospital's computer network that the tissue he had just examined was strongly suspicious of malignant melanoma (amelanotic).

Dr. Elie forwarded this to the Ear, Nose and Throat department of the Navy Hospital at Jacksonville. Then he made some more slides of the tissue and sent them to Bethesda, Maryland, to the Armed Forces Institute of Pathology—the AFIP. He wanted confirmation of his suspicions from this world-renowned organization.

Until the sample was confirmed as malignant melanoma by the AFIP, well, maybe this was all one big mistake. "Strongly suspicious of" is not a definite. Maybe Dr. Elie had made a mistake. Maybe it was a harmless cyst on my ear after all. Until the AFIP came back with the specific results of their analysis, which consisted of far more complex staining of the tissues than was possible by Dr. Elie, I was in limbo. I was told that the AFIP would be handling my biopsy specimen as a priority and it would take no more than a week for their report to get back to Dr. Fischer.

This allowed me a margin of hope. Maybe the good doctor Elie had made a mistake. Maybe his eyes were playing tricks on him when he looked through his microscope. Maybe he was wrong. That's where my hope lay. (Okay, maybe there was a little denial mixed in.) Boy, oh boy, did I ever hope—and pray—that it was all a terrible mistake.

Or maybe it was just a simple case of mistaken identity, because Lord knows, with a wife and six-year-old twins, I was way too young and way too healthy to be at death's door. Maybe the tissue that Dr. Elie had biopsied had come from someone else's body and had been mislabeled.

Yes, there was still a chance that the Jacksonville Navy Hospital's pathology department was wrong. Perhaps it was just a harmless fatty cyst after all. Hope. You've got to love it. It is all-important. But when hope and denial merge and become blurred, well, now you've got the start of a real problem. And this started to become a problem for me as I drove home, trying to figure out exactly how to break this latest news to Peggy, Brian, and Christie. Would I put on a big smile and be unrealistically hopeful, or would I put on my game face and say to myself, "No way, not me, not Bill Goss," or would I just be angry at the world? Like most people, I would end up doing all of those things at one time or another throughout this ordeal.

A close friend of mine, Rudy Ruettiger, the inspiring real-life Notre Dame football player behind the blockbuster movie *Rudy*, learned how to use his anger in a constructive way. He used it to inspire himself and to prove to the people who mocked him and told him to give up on his dream that they were wrong. Dead wrong. Even though he graduated number two in his high school class (number two from the bottom, that is), Rudy ended up both graduating from and playing football for the Fighting Irish of Notre Dame. He just had to put his heart and soul into it, even after he was diagnosed with dyslexia, which made it very tough for him to read and study all that was required of him at a great university like Notre Dame. Rudy just had to remain focused on his dream and shake off the difficulties, struggles, and obstacles that are always placed in front of giant goals and spectacular dreams. After all, if we didn't have challenges, our dreams would all be achieved, and they would be ordinary, no longer spectacular. Rudy just had to make sure the words "I quit" never crossed his lips. They could cross his mind, but never his lips.

I recalled the movie as I drove home. I hadn't met Rudy yet, but figured I would do the same as that tough little guy I admired. I would not quit. I would reach my dream. And I would not have a dream that was crazy or nearly impossible or unattainable. I would keep it simple. And so this became my goal and my dream: to see my children graduate sixth grade at Paterson Elementary School. They were in first grade now. If I was successful at achieving this goal it would mean I had blasted through the five-year cancer survival milestone in a blaze of glory.

No matter what it took, I would be there at Christie and Brian's graduation. With cancer, surgical removal of the primary and even secondary tumors often has the highest precedence in the early stages of treating this disease. Without a doubt, if the AFIP confirmed that my biopsy was malignant melanoma, my left ear was history. It would have to go. And I would want it to go. Even if my surgeons had to surgically remove every limb of my body, I would do it, if that was necessary for me to be at Christie and Brian's graduation. Nothing was going to stop me from attending it. Nothing.

When I pulled into our driveway, Peggy met me outside.

"Bill, the kids don't need to know a thing now. Let's really think this thing through before we tell them anything about you having cancer."

"Good plan, Peg," I said, having arrived home without even a clue of how or what I would tell my family, except that it would be the truth, as much as I knew at the time.

I explained to Peggy what Dr. Fischer had told me about the gravely serious situation I—we—were in. Peggy was amazing in her simplicity and her strength.

"Bill, you'll overcome this challenge, just like you've overcome all the other challenges that have come your way." She was right. I had overcome a lot of adversity. Maybe all the other things that had happened to me were simply to prepare me for the greatest challenge of all. Cancer.

I called my father, a former manager at a life insurance company, who, along with my mother, urged me to go outside the Navy medical system and get a nonmilitary second opinion *now.* I took Dad's advice to heart. I never professed to be a rocket scientist (I'll leave that to my brother-in-law, Danny, who truly is a NASA rocket scientist), but one of my strengths has been to seek and recognize when I was getting good advice, and more important, to follow through on it.

That day, a friend who had learned of my situation called to tell me that he could help me get an appointment to be evaluated by the Tumor Review Board at the University of Florida's Shands Hospital. Remarkably, this board just happened to be scheduled for the following morning in Gainesville, Florida. What luck. Sometimes luck and speed and timing are everything, especially with cancer. Every second that ticks by could be that very second, that terribly discrete fraction of a moment when your primary tumor decides to start shedding additional cancer cells into your bloodstream, which can then metastasize into a secondary tumor in another part of your body, dramatically complicating the treatment.

At that moment, I believed I had only one tumor. A second tumor was definitely not something I wanted to think about. One highly malignant tumor just an inch from my brain was more than enough for me to deal with, thank you—and it was the reason why I wanted to move ahead so quickly and aggressively with my treatment. I wanted desperately to beat any new tumors to the punch. I saw speed and appropriate and aggressive treatment as essential to surviving this thing . . . if I had cancer at all (there's that hope and denial thing again). My tumor's true identity had not yet been confirmed by the Armed Forces Institute of Pathology, so, in some small way, I was still holding out for a miracle.

What's a tumor review board? It's a small group of doctors from a variety of medical disciplines (in my case, ear, nose and throat; radiology; oncology; pathology, etc.) who get together to look at specific data and examine patients associated with some of the more atypical cancer cases. These doctors then collectively offer a recommendation to the patient and to the patient's primary care physician as to what they think is the best course of treatment. Going through a tumor review board was like getting ten or more second opinions—extremely valuable information.

Like a good Navy pilot, I wanted to know more about the enemy than the enemy knew about me. If I didn't discover how to take charge of my cancer it was certainly going to take charge of Bill Goss. It seemed like my tumor was trying to take on a life of its own. Maybe it already had. . . .

The two-hour drive from my home in Orange Park to Shands Hospital gave me additional time to think—and pray—and hope—and deny. I remembered the phone call I had with Dr. Cassisi, head of the Shands Tumor Review Board, the night before.

Dr. Cassisi said, "Lieutenant Commander Goss, don't forget—the most important thing for you to do tomorrow is to bring with you the microscope slides of your tumor. Don't waste your time driving down here unless you bring them with you. Without those slides, we won't be able to tell you a thing. Without those slides, we won't be able to help you."

Thank God that Anton van Leeuwenhoek invented the microscope in Holland more than three hundred years ago—imagine how many lives that guy has saved by now. It didn't help that my hospital had misplaced the slides of my biopsy, but thankfully Dr. Elie was able to find an extra set for me to take to Shands in Gainesville just in time.

When doctors discuss cancer, particularly *your* cancer, what they see under a microscope on your biopsy slides is a matter of life and death. Unfortunately, what the doctors at Shands saw on my slides was not life. At least not what we consider good life. It was not a fatty cyst. It was something bad. Something really, really bad.

After the six-hour tumor review board was over, one older doctor privately shared with me his personal thoughts on his findings. "Son," he said, "it's time to get your life in order." When I told him that I felt my life was already in fine order, he looked at me, shook his head, and walked away. What a disastrous bedside manner. A person's desire to fight the cancer battle—to have hope—should not be dashed into tiny pieces by anyone, and certainly not by some allegedly compassionate medical professional whose only advice is to prepare your will.

Throughout my ordeal, the rest of the doctors and nurses I dealt with were exemplary—absolutely beyond reproach. It's amazing how the human mind works. With all the incredible medical professionals who touched me and helped me to heal—and I remember them all very well—recalling that one callous remark still raises the hairs on the back of my neck.

In retrospect, that doctor might have touched a nerve of mine so raw that for all I know, I might have used my anger— anger directed at him—*just to prove him wrong* by staying alive. I think it might be the only time I used my anger in a positive way to fight cancer. Remarkably, I had very little anger at anybody or anything else. Just that one insensitive doctor. Of course, he might have thought he was only being honest, not insensitive.

The day I went through the tumor review board at Shands, I was going through another review board that was just as important, only I wasn't there. My tumor was sent there in my place to represent me. This review board was at the Armed Forces Institute of Pathology, one of the largest and most advanced military medical complexes in the world. Located in Bethesda, Maryland, the AFIP had just completed a very tricky chemical staining of another set of microscopic slides that had an ultra-thin sliver of my tumor on it.

I guess if you can slice something thin enough, there's enough of it to go around to everyone. I had to keep reminding myself that although it was a tumor and not a very nice thing, it still was pure Goss tissue through and through. But it was Goss tissue that just refused to die. That is the definition of cancer—cells that divide indefinitely and out of control, cells that just don't age, or wear out, or die, like all living cells are supposed to do sooner or later. Cancer is really a general term for a group of more than one hundred diseases characterized by the uncontrolled growth and spread of abnormal cells. When cells divide when new ones aren't needed, they form a mass of excess tissue called a tumor. Tumors can be benign (noncancerous) or malignant (cancerous). Benign tumors generally stay put while malignant tumors tend to invade and damage nearby and distant tissues and organs.

Both boards, the one at Shands Gainesville and the one at the Armed Forces Institute of Pathology in Bethesda, came up with the same stinking dirty rotten conclusion. Cancer. And not just cancer, but a highly malignant form that was far deeper beneath my skin than your normal, already dangerous melanoma.

The severity of skin cancer is determined by how many layers of epidermis the tumor has grown down through in its attempt to seek out a greater blood supply to feed it, such as the squamous skin cell layer, and then, beneath that, the basal skin cell layer. The first two forms of skin cancer—squamous cell (200,000 new cases each year) and basal cell (800,000 new cases each year)—are unpleasant and sometimes terribly disfiguring, but these forms of skin cancer are usually not fatal. Remember, I said *usually* not fatal. They still can kill.

But, by and large, malignant melanoma is much more malignant than other forms of skin cancer, hence the name malignant melanoma. Usually quite easy to spot and detect in its earliest stages, once a melanoma mole has seated deeply into your skin tissue and sent its roots down through your inner (dermis) layer of skin, reaching a greater blood supply, it offers a poor prognosis for long-term survival. Like mine.

Malignant melanoma is a cancer of melanocytes, those pigment-producing cells spread throughout our skin that make the melanin (skin pigment) that causes our skin to tan when exposed to radiation from the sun. The more naturally occurring melanin in our skin, the more protected we are from the sun's radiation. That is why people from equatorial areas of the world have evolved to have darker skin than northern Europeans—to protect them from the intense radiation effects of the sun on continents near the equator.

When cells are struck by too much radiation, it can cause the molecular structure of the cells' DNA to mutate. These mutant cells sometimes are able to survive—though mutants of anything usually don't—and then they begin to divide uncontrollably. Instead of dying like regular cells normally do after they have divided fifty to one hundred times, cancer cells seem to live forever, crowding out the healthy cells. If you have a powerful immune response, your immune system should gobble those mutated cells up right away, well before they multiply into a deadly multicellular growth, commonly called a malignant tumor.

But sometimes even a healthy immune system can't keep up with aggressively proliferating cancer cells. Every case is unique. In its earliest stages, cancer growth depends on how aggressive the tumor is and on how powerful a person's immune response is to that type of tumor.

Generally, in the case of malignant melanoma, if the tumor starts to reach a good blood supply to feed its growth, the cancerous melanocytes begin to go wild with growth, dramatically overproducing melanin, which is why it typically shows up one day as either a dark or multishaded new mole or as a rapidly changing existing mole.

I, however, had a rare, one-in-a-thousand form of this disease: amelanotic malignant melanoma. It had the same deadly characteristics as normal melanoma, except there was no overproduction of melanin, so the skin on my left ear was perfectly normal-looking except for the bump. And bumps under normal-appearing skin are very characteristic of the kinds of harmless cysts commonly found on human ears. Initially, the bump on my ear likely would have been misdiagnosed by almost any doctor, even an experienced dermatologist. Without discoloration of the skin, the bump on my left ear didn't appear even remotely like a deadly melanoma. Not to anybody. It's something that most doctors have never seen, even after years of medical practice.

The real kicker was this: The one or two medical books that mentioned the existence of amelanotic malignant melanoma stated that it showed up only at metastatic, or secondary sites. Malignant melanoma was virtually never without melanin at the site of the *primary* tumor. What did this mean? That the little melanin-free tumor on my ear was unlikely to be the only one I had. It was better than even money that I had another, melanotic tumor somewhere else inside me.

One of the things I learned about how to deal with the challenges of cancer is that procedurally things seem to follow a definite order with indefinite periods of time between each stage. Some things I was unable to control, like how fast the AFIP got back to me with their confirmation of the pathology of my disease. Other things I could control, like how much information about my disease I could assimilate and process so that I could make faster and, I hoped, smarter decisions to speed us to the next very likely step: surgery to reduce the potential for metastatic spread of the tumor.

While waiting for my surgery to be scheduled, I went to the library to research my disease. This was a subject I obviously wanted to understand with as much depth as possible—with more depth and knowledge than even my doctors. Whatever the survival rate was, I was going to claim it as my own. But I had to know the real data about this disease, not a rough estimate. As a Navy pilot I wanted to know more about my adversary than my adversary knew about me. Now that my adversary was inside me, I had to get inside my adversary. To me, it was that simple. Maybe it was my years of training and experiences as a Navy pilot that made it that simple for me. But getting that experience had not been "that simple" at all.

We are the culmination of our experiences and our basic genetic makeup. And probably some people are better prepared than others, first, at not getting cancer, and second, at winning the fight against cancer if they do get it. I certainly wasn't in the first group. I was hoping—and praying—I was in the second group.

I was going to take all my life's experiences and use them in my battle against cancer. I found a quiet spot in a rarely frequented corner of the Orange Park Library to continue my research on a disease I'd known almost nothing about just a few days earlier. I started by looking up the word *malignant* in the dictionary. I knew roughly what it meant. But now—now that it was being used in reference to something happening inside *my* body, the word suddenly took on a whole new meaning. I felt it was time for me to know *exactly* how "malignant" was defined.

Here's the dictionary's definition: "Deadly; tending to produce death, as in a disease or tumor." Okay, that's kind of what I'd figured.

Next, I checked out the *Merck Manual*, widely regarded as the bible of modern medicine. Under the heading "Malignant Melanoma," I found the following very chilling words: "May spread so rapidly that it will be fatal within months of recognition." Not what I wanted to read, but it definitely confirmed why the doctors had been looking at me so forlornly.

Since my pathology report stated I had an "unknown primary cancer," I looked up that phrase as well. The words frightened me further: "These patients account for 0.5% to 7% of all cancer patients—survival in patients with an unknown primary cancer is generally poor—median is 3–4 months—metastatic melanoma cannot be cured at present." This was devastating information to receive in any form. Maybe burying my head in the sand would have been a smarter thing for me to do than to read this crap. I started feeling uneasy and alone, even queasy.

At least on paper, the odds for my survival were abysmal. I buried my face in my arm, hidden from view, deep in the recesses of our town library, feeling sick with grief at the thought of leaving Peggy and the kids to find their way through life without me.

I guess I'm just like any other person, I thought. Long on faith and hope one minute, short on it the next. Now that I had gone to the effort to cram all that cancer data and specific melanoma statistics into my brain, I desperately wanted that information out of there.

Oh, yes, my brain. I had other things to think about as well. With my tumor only an inch from my brain, there was a great concern that it had already spread there. If that was the case, my doctors said, all curative treatments would stop. All they could do then would be to try to kill the pain. This is called "palliative treatment." It means all hope for a cure is gone, so let's focus on as gentle a death as possible.

Thankfully, melanoma treatments have improved somewhat since then, but at the time, brain melanoma was considered inoperable and incurable. Obviously I did not want palliative treatment. I wanted a cure, so I prayed fervently that my brain scan would show up negative for any kind of metastatic lesions. According to some doctors, if such a thing happened I would be extraordinarily lucky, considering all the aspects of my case.

I was scheduled for an immediate CAT scan of my brain, lungs, heart, and liver. What's a CAT scan? Also referred to as a CT scan, the acronym CAT stands for computerized axial tomography. One of the greatest technological advances in modern medicine since the discovery of X rays, the CAT scan combines multiple low-dose X rays rotated around the axis of your body (that's where the word *axial* comes from) with the powerful processing ability and memory of the modern computer chip. Through the very clever combination of these technologies, a CAT scan of the human body can provide a doctor with a multicolor three-dimensional visualization of the internal organs, at a near-microscopic level. After review by a qualified radiologist—an M.D. who specializes in evaluating X-ray and other radiology-related medical data—a phenomenal diagnostic tool is now at the hands of your physician, especially for quick assessment of internal injuries and for early detection and progression of cancer.

Some of the other scanning procedures I would ultimately be exposed to over the course of my treatment (besides an annual chest X ray looking for malignant melanoma metastasis to my lungs) were MRIs (magnetic resonance imaging), bone scans, and PET scans (positron emission tomography).

(CAT scans and PET scans—soon a radiologist with a touch of marketing genius will discover a technology so that the acronym DOG scan can somehow enter the medical lingo. What could it possibly stand for. . . . digital orbital gonad scan?)

In any case, if the CAT scans were negative for tumors, that would be great news, although microscopic cancer cells that had lodged in any of my organs or lymph nodes would be undetectable and would likely show up eventually. But even if that were the case, a lack of visible tumors in this set of CAT scans could potentially buy me some time. Time to see my kids graduate the sixth grade.

Peggy, tremendously loving and supportive throughout this ordeal, listened when I had something to say and stayed close by my side when I didn't. She handled phone calls I did not want or need to take, and answered tough and sometimes rude or impertinent questions from others with style and grace. She made my favorite meals. If she cried or worried, which I know she must have at times, she courageously avoided doing it around the children and me. She not only kept a stiff upper lip, she somehow kept her cool and her dignity as she prepared to face the storm. She's really an extraordinarily strong person in so many ways.

Of course, I didn't share with her everything I read; I didn't want to depress her. A little selfishly, I knew I had to keep her as upbeat and positive as possible. If she became deeply depressed while I was trying to beat back the cancer, it would make it immeasurably harder to emerge victorious.

Ultimately, Peggy proved to be perfect in every way imaginable as the days rapidly closed in on my surgery. But even with a perfect spouse, dealing with cancer—particularly at those times when there is not a lot of hope in the equation—is sometimes still an excruciatingly lonely proposition.

Brian and Christie still didn't have a clue. We weren't sure as to the best way to be honest with them without scaring them half to death. How were we going to tell them that Daddy was sick and was soon going to the hospital for a very big operation? And that when he came home Daddy was probably going to be kind of scary-looking for a while, but that he would somehow get better, especially if we gave him lots of hugs and kisses and we didn't worry too much about how he looked? And there was good news for them, too . . . Daddy would probably be home a lot more to play with them.

We told them many stories of other crazy things that had happened to me in my past and how I had always somehow come through those challenges better and stronger than before. We told them that this is how things always worked out for Daddy. Those crazy stories from my past—especially the ones that included my boyhood friends—comforted Christie and Brian and even made them laugh. We also said a lot of simple little prayers together, especially at dinner.

At the time, I was working for the admiral in charge of most of the Navy's facilities in the southeastern United States. He was a good man and one of the Navy's most senior pilots. Like all smart flag officers, this admiral had his own under-ground network of information. Apparently, the commanding officer of the Navy hospital, who served under the admiral in the chain of command, gave the admiral a courtesy call regard-ing me and my predicament. The hospital commanding officer must have given him a very bleak prognosis because the next day he grabbed me by the arm and pulled me into his office. He told me that the most important thing right now was that I got better. He wanted me to spend my time with my wife and kids and to focus on one task—recovery.

It was an important conversation and helped reduce stresses in my life that would not have helped me get better. Being told not to worry about work, but to focus only on get-ting well, is a message more people need to hear when they get seriously ill. Wherever you are now, Admiral, thank you. In some ways I feel like I needed that very direct and explicit order from you to get better.

But it was no bed of optimism for me. Believe me, I still had worries. Very late one night, unable to sleep, I gently climbed out of bed, careful not to wake Peggy, who really needed her sleep, too. I went outside and stood, head back, under the immensity of the stars. Staring deeply into an indigo sky filled with countless stars, out loud I implored, "If you are listening to my prayers, to my heart, please, please show me a sign." I waited, face pointed to the heavens. After a while I finally said to myself, "This is stupid. What am I really waiting for—an answer?"

Just as I started to turn back to my house, the largest meteor I've ever seen, a blinding white fireball, torched across the sky to the south, as though it were beckoning me to follow. I fell onto our back-porch step and for a good five seconds watched the blazing streak of the meteor tail slowly twinkle into oblivion.

Face in hands, I started to cry. For God to have waited until the exact moment in which my shallow faith failed before lighting my way was an incredibly powerful message for me to receive at that point in space and time. Suddenly I no longer felt the horrendous anguish of feeling alone and separate from the universe. I now knew the universe was part of me and I was part of it. It was like I had been lost forever in a darkened room, then suddenly my fingers happened upon the light switch and everything became crystal clear.

I now knew that some incredible force was with me and always had been. I had been reminded at the perfect time that God is real, prayer is powerful, and faith, even in small amounts, means everything.

With renewed hope and a fired-up human spirit, the next day I went in for a CAT scan. First they had me drink about four large containers of what looked like a vanilla milkshake but unfortunately tasted like liquid chalk. Then an IV was stuck into my arm that caused an instant and very unusual chill to course through my veins.

I put on my game face. After all, I was a brave Navy pilot. Keep thinking positive, I said to myself, while laid flat out in the claustrophobic tomblike enclosure so characteristic of older CAT scan machines, the steril smell of rubbing alcohol filling the narrow space. If you've ever been in a CAT scan machine, you know that the only parts of your body you might be able to get a good look at are your hands. I looked at my left hand and noticed it was shaking like a leaf. Self, I said to myself, your brain may be brave, but your hand is terrified.

Suddenly, like a fist right between the eyes, it dawned on me that I was looking at an important symbol—my five fingers. I think it must have been my wedding ring that triggered this line of thought. That ring represented fourteen years of being married to Peggy; we'd eloped in Pensacola, Florida, right before I started Navy pilot training. My love for Peggy and our children was like a tail hook tethering me to life. And just as suddenly, I realized that there were four other important life-lines that together held me securely, just as my five fingers had once cradled my babies' heads. What I now refer to as my Five Fs of Fulfillment had gotten me through so many earlier escapes and challenges. I now saw that, as essential as these five Fs had been in my past, they were critical to my success in the future. Critical as I faced the greatest challenge of my life—cancer.

The five Fs are: Family, Friends, Faith, Focus, and Fun.

My family had gotten me through much during childhood, starting with my not talking until age five, which, as you can imagine, put quite a label on me for a spell. Also I was a natural recluse, much more at home alone in the woods with animals, especially snakes, than anywhere else. That, combined with the uncoordinated clumsiness that comes from being the only leftie in a family of eight, probably set me apart from other children rather quickly, though my grandmother finally got me to write with my right hand "like normal people."

As a leftie, I was a very short-lived disaster on the Little League baseball field, much to the quiet dismay of my father, a former (right-handed) pitcher on the Seton Hall University baseball team who used the G.I. Bill to get a master's degree in education. (Dad earned the rank of chief petty officer in the Coast Guard in record time. He was directly involved in three major amphibious invasions in the Pacific during WW II— Okinawa, Guam, and Leyte. There aren't many people still around like my father—I consider him a true hero.)

But, with a lot of love, patience, and occasional corporal punishment, combined with a major surge of testosterone in seventh grade, I started to find my way into the world of sports, girls, and even, occasionally, school. I think I even made up for being such a lousy baseball player in my father's eyes after he watched me play varsity middle linebacker on our high school football team and also start to excel in boxing and wrestling.

We kids were blessed with an equally strong mother and father. Barbara and Eugene Goss individually and collectively demonstrated a sense of values I took with me into my own marriage. There were always a lot of strong feelings in our household. Strong love, strong opinions—and strong differences of opinion. Through it all, my three sisters and two brothers helped me immensely in countless ways.

My eldest sister, Mimi, Goss kid number one, probably got stuck doing more than her fair share of baby-sitting me, even though she is only five years older than I. Always a great student, Mimi taught me that if you applied yourself to your studies, you would do well in school. She was also the first of us to travel the world on her own, which strongly influenced my wanderlust as well. The mother of one son, Mimi earned a doctorate in communications and is now a professor at Harvard's Kennedy School of Government.

Four years older than I, my eldest brother, Bob, taught me that if you wanted money, you had to go out and get a job and just do the work. From junior high school on, I never remember Bobby not having a paying job outside the home. He really taught me how to stretch a dollar—and how to appreciate fine rock 'n' roll. The father of two boys, Bob finessed his way into a successful career on Wall Street.

Two years older than I, brother Larry taught me to be quick on my feet. A superbly built athlete, an excellent wrestler, and very popular with the ladies, Larry engaged me in countless physical battles, some friendly, some not so friendly, but every one of them made me tougher, faster, and stronger. Larry now owns and runs several businesses in Rhode Island and is the father of two daughters and a son.

One year younger than I, sister Greta suffered the humiliation of my dating some of her girlfriends in high school. Highly energetic and very creative, Greta is the mother of an animal-loving son and an adopted daughter from Russia. Greta is now a highly regarded interior designer in Montclair, New Jersey.

And five years younger than I is sister Jackie. Jackie is the favorite of all of us because we all remember how cute she was as a baby. She was absolutely adorable—and still is. People are drawn to Jackie not only because she is beautiful but because she is smart and has a great sense of humor. The mother of a girl and a boy, Jackie is a successful realtor in Austin, Texas.

I think the greatest thing the six Goss siblings accomplished—a testament to the self-reliance, work ethic, and, yes, even wanderlust that my parents ingrained first into Mimi, and then into the rest of us—was that we not only graduated college but, more important, paid our own way, which is how we all came to appreciate the true value of advanced education. Every college-credit hour a Goss kid earned toward a degree not only represented hard work in the classroom, it usually represented even harder work at a part-time job to pay for it. We learned both the value of an education and the value of a dollar at the same time. I still consider it one of the most valuable lessons a kid can learn.

On top of that, none of us attended college near home, except for me, and that requires an explanation. After a year at the University of Arizona in Tucson, then two years traveling around the world building underwater weapons while a mine man in the Navy, I returned home to New Jersey to finish college at Rutgers University, before becoming a Navy pilot and setting out all over the world again.

But as a general rule in the Goss household, when you turned eighteen you were legally considered an adult and no one was accountable for you but you. You were strongly—very strongly—encouraged to go out and hit the road on your own and oh, by the way, come back with a college degree. My siblings and I all welcomed and proudly met that challenge.

The close relationship I have with my family has been an integral part of my successful fight against cancer. The powerful network of family extends even further to my brothers- and sisters-in-law, my father-in-law, aunts and uncles, nieces and nephews, and cousins. There is a lot of good blood between us—and a supercharged immune system depends on good blood. Good blood that is recharged often.

But even more important is the family relationship I have

with Peggy and our twins, Brian and Christie. My immediate family, combined with the houseful of animals that make up the menagerie at Goss Central in Florida, is what my life is really about. I'll go into a lot of detail about them later, especially that little ball of fur that fell from the sky and into my heart, but collectively they unite to make Family, the first F in the Five Fs of Fulfillment.

The second F is Friends. Where would we be without our friends? I was lucky enough to be born and grow up in the same relatively small town in New Jersey. Even though I moved away at age eighteen, I am still blessed to have numerous close buddies from as far back as kindergarten. I talk with them at least once a month and they are very supportive and understanding, especially regarding cancer, probably because several of them have lost at least one parent from it. When you can't talk to your family—and let's face it, sometimes you can't—nothing tops the listening ear and sage advice of a very close friend.

The third F is Faith. If you don't believe in a higher power, then you are forced to believe that everything that happens in the world is either a random event or totally dependent on you—unsettling concepts for most people, myself included. My faith has saved me so many times, believing that someone or something is looking out for me just comes naturally now— though an occasional recharge from a timely meteor never hurts. The important thing I've learned about prayer is not to ask for anything. Instead, just give thanks for all the tools you have already been blessed with and then go to work using those tools to make your dreams and goals a reality. God truly helps those who help themselves—and help others. Audrey Hepburn once said that we were blessed with two hands. One hand to take care of ourselves, the other to take care of others.

The fourth F is Focus. You must concentrate most on the goal or dream you most want to accomplish or achieve. Like a magnifying glass turning diffuse sunlight into an intense beam that ignites anything in its path, you must sometimes take all your energy—and sometimes all the energy of your family and your friends—to make truly wondrous and miraculous things happen. It's how the Amish farmers raise a barn in just a day: focus of energy, talent, spirit, and faith.

And the fifth F, like the last finger on your hand, is Fun. Without fun, life just doesn't seem worth living. Fun and laughter recharge the human spirit, revitalize all your different loves, and positively charge the immune system. Fun makes you want to go the extra mile. Making money should be fun, but money should also be used for having fun and for helping other people enjoy a better quality of life. Giving freely and abundantly is fun. One of the most significant reasons I want to live for a very long time is that I want to have as much fun as I possibly can with my family and friends and to give freely and generously to those less fortunate than myself. Why? Because I enjoy it—because it's fun.

The Five Fs of Fulfillment. That what I learned while I was getting my brain scan for cancer. As for that brain scan: After it was over, I asked the technician, a wonderful woman named Kevin who keeps a photograph of a cat receiving an X ray on her door, if she would let me look at her computer monitor to see the images I knew were instantly available to her. She agreed, and the technology suddenly before my eyes was truly a marvel to behold.

She zoomed in on a portion of the CAT scan and enlarged it so I could see in great detail, explaining all the various parts and how they should look under normal and then under not-so-normal conditions. Although a trained radiologist, not

Kevin, would evaluate my scans as to whether they were positive or negative for mets—medical lingo for cancerous metastatic lesions—I sensed from Kevin's friendly demeanor that at least she was comfortable with the images she was looking at. And she had seen thousands and thousands of CAT scans over her career.

Just like Dr. Elie, who showed me my pathology slides under his microscope and explained his conclusions to me in detail, Kevin had great respect and compassion for the people with serious problems who stepped into her world for a time, especially when she could see that they had a sincere desire to learn what was going on inside their bodies so they could live longer, healthier, happier lives. A few days later, Kevin did a CAT scan of my torso, paying particular attention to my lungs, heart, liver, and lymphatic system—lymph nodes—looking, always looking, for mets. Thankfully, there were none.

(I have to admit, looking at the computer image of my entire body in front of her, well, it was kind of embarrassing: The images were so damned good. Shrinkage, if you know what I mean.)

A few days later, after the radiologists reviewed my CAT scans and reported no obvious mets in my brain or in my abdominal cavity, I was finally scheduled for surgery.

When he was in his late nineties, his frail and shrunken body having become like a prison to his extraordinary human spirit, my grandfather Charles "Pop" Dacey said something that truly defined who he was.

"Billy, it's not the pace of life that ever bothered me, it's that sudden stop at the end." I believe Pop welcomed—with his typical sense of humor—his death, so that his human spirit could again explode into Mother Nature and the universe, with the energy of a million teenagers.

My generous grandmother Frances "Nana" Dacey, who died in her nineties, not long before Pop, shared the same view of how youthful the human spirit can be, despite the condition of the body that contains it. Nana told my sister Mimi, when she was in her twenties and my grandmother was in her late seventies, "When I look in the mirror, I am always shocked, because I am expecting to see someone who looks like you, not a little old lady."

These are just a few examples of how my grandparents provided me with invaluable insights into the nature and meaning of the human spirit. What meaning did this have regarding my life and with what I was going through with cancer? A lot. I was thirty-eight years old. I not only felt strong and looked strong, I was strong. I had a beautiful wife and kids I was committed to being with for a long time to come. I still had a huge personal mission ahead of me—to fulfill my obligations as a father and as a husband. Unlike my amazing grandparents, my spirit and my body were in step with each other, ready to move forward in perfect sync in my quest for many more years of healthy life. But I had to take that first step—radical cancer surgery—and take it quick, if I was going to pull off another of my great escapes.

So, with near delight, I was scheduled to have my left ear lopped off, along with the salivary gland, jugular vein, trapezoidal muscle, and 150 to 200 lymph nodes from the left side of my face, shoulder, and neck. To me, getting scheduled for this surgery was good news. Very very good news.

Why? Because if the radiologists had found signs of mets in my CAT scans, particularly metastatic lesions in any of my vital organs like my brain, heart, lungs, or liver, the hospital would probably not have scheduled me for surgery.

According to one doctor, "What would have been the point?"

So I considered myself lucky. I got psyched up and pumped up and prepared to do battle. Armed with my newly discovered Five Fs of Fulfillment, I was ready for the extensive cancer surgery.

With a powerfully recharged human spirit that I was certain was also helping to powerfully recharge my immune system, I started to look forward to the challenge that lay before me. Another great adventure in my life—a spectacular continuation of my human spirit's journey. Not a journey to just survive cancer. But a journey to thrive—*thrive*—in the very face of it.

3

Tapping in to Mother Nature

A large amount of research has gone into the powerful bond that exists between humans and animals. Recently, a lot has been written about the subject, particularly by a great friend of mine in Idaho, Dr. Marty Becker, the veterinary contributor to ABC TV's *Good Morning America* and author of the bestseller *The Healing Power of Pets*. In my opinion, Marty Becker has done more than any other person I know to prove that our greatest healers, teachers, and heroes have fur, feathers, or four legs.

Other people with heightened awareness, particularly Native Americans, have demonstrated similar connections between enhanced human healing and animal contact. It's been demonstrated in the tremendous power of horse therapy in helping autistic children connect better with the world. And certain positive and powerful changes have been documented among people with mental and physical challenges when they swim with bottle-nosed dolphins. Sometimes it seems like these people's batteries have been recharged or they've been given a new lease on life just moments after they have been put in the company of some gentle animals, in a field full of wildflowers, or under the shade of a three-hundred-foot tall redwood.

I believe with all my heart that a bond exists between all God's creations. As a boy I would climb a tall tree and lose myself in rapture as I watched powerful raptors like the mighty goshawk soar in the thermals along the mountainside near our home. Watching them sail effortlessly among the clouds, like angels with feathers, I yearned to fly like them, soaring into the heavens at a moment's notice. The inspiration and desire to fly as a Navy pilot certainly, in large part, came from the splendid treetop view I had of those birds migrating along South Mountain behind our home.

But even more, being in the woods and connecting with nature always made me feel that no matter what happened to me, I would somehow make it through life without too much difficulty. Alone with Mother Nature, I was calm. I felt at peace with myself much more in the woods than I did when at school or in our home. As a boy, I would beg to sleep outside, under the canopy of the stars, ever on the lookout for a bat, an owl, a whippoorwill, or some other mysterious creature of the night sky.

Thirty years later, in the weeks between my initial cancer diagnosis and the twelve hours of surgery, I again took solace in nature. I again took time to reflect on my life and the things that were important to me, and how they all fit into the bigger picture—the much bigger picture that encompassed all of life itself: Mother Nature.

Peggy and I created an arboretumlike setting around our home on historic Fleming Island in Orange Park, a town that borders the southwest corner of Jacksonville, Florida. Orange Park was named after the large groves it was known for, before all the citrus trees were killed during a lengthy winter freeze in the early 1900s.

I've always loved the lush natural beauty of Florida. Evidently so did Ponce de León. When he first walked the land in 1513 in what is now St. Augustine, just thirty miles south of us, he found it so beautiful he called it La Florida, meaning "land of flowers."

Peggy and I bought a large red-brick home on a small private road in the woods that dead ends on a part of the St. Johns River, which is about four miles wide. Together with the twelve other families with whom we share our little street, we built a spectacular nature walk and dock that first winds for one thousand feet through a beautiful cypress wetlands area, and then out into the St. Johns River for another thousand feet, all to better appreciate nature in all its glory.

First you might ask, "So what's so historic about historic Fleming Island?" Good question. South of our dock, a mile or two down the shoreline, you can barely see the remains of what was once another family's dock and pier. Remarkably, the wood pilings that are still visible at low tide are more than 150 years old, a testament to the cypress wood used back then, wood so impervious to termites and any form of decay that it was also the wood of choice in the construction of the ocean-going vessels of the day.

As I've heard the story told, in 1837 young Margaret Seton

married the widowed Lewis Fleming, who had inherited the island from his father. Over the next twenty years, Margaret and Lewis raised ten children in an enormous wood-framed plantation house that backed up to the St. Johns River. During the more temperate months, when the workload on their plantation slowed down, they would sometimes have as many as fifty houseguests. For recreation, they played golf on a nine-hole course they built just down the road from where our house now stands. Hibernia Links was one of the first golf courses in North America. Men played golf in suits and ties. Women played in long, billowy dresses. Rumor has it that Margaret Seton was a pretty damn good player. But it wasn't all fun and games.

Early one morning their house was raided and burned to the ground by Indians. Amazingly, the entire Fleming family somehow escaped into the woods unharmed. Over the course of the next few years, Margaret and Lewis completely rebuilt their rambling three-story home from the ground up. Soon after that, three of their sons went off to fight in the Civil War. Standing on the cypress dock directly behind their home, Margaret would carefully observe the Federal gunboats as they patrolled up and down the river.

One of their sons, Seton, was captured and held in a prisoner-of-war camp in the North. Using the skills he'd learned as a boy fishing for bream from their sturdy cypress dock, he caught rats at night in his prison cell to stave off the starvation that eventually killed so many of his fellow POWs. Luckily, he survived to see his family again and to even fish with them again on the long cypress dock behind their home.

With her indomitable spirit and character, Margaret also funded the construction of a tiny Episcopal church right down the road from us on Fleming Island. Sadly, the first service held at St. Margaret's was a funeral in 1878—the funeral of the little church's inspiring benefactor, Margaret Seton Fleming.

Now, besides the beautiful old church, all that remains of the Flemings is a grove of giant oaks that Margaret planted. That and the broken posts of their cypress dock, reaching up from the St. Johns River like ghosts clawing their way to the heavens.

Thankfully, the dock and nature walk we had constructed was brand new, made of pressure-treated wood rather than the prohibitively expensive cypress. It had neither a colorful nor a haunted past. It was just commencing its own, unique history. And it was completed just in time for my family and me to start using it to tap in to the incredibly powerful healing forces I felt certain to connect with simply by spending time outdoors, under both the sun and the moon, the clouds and the stars. The end of our dock was—and still is—a wonderful place for reflection. This is especially true when watching the sun rise in the morning mist, with the snowy egrets, great blue herons, diving ospreys, patrolling pelicans, and an occasional bald eagle reminding this newly grounded Navy pilot of the miracle and pure joy of flight.

Every walk down to the end of our dock is an entirely different experience because the tides constantly change with the moon's orbit. And regardless of tidal effects, approximately 3.5 billion gallons of St. Johns River water flow by our dock every day, northward, from Lake George to the Atlantic Ocean.

With the changes in tides comes changes in smells. Sometimes in the springtime, our nature walk smells as sweet as honey from all the blooming wildflowers. In the summer, the vegetation gets as thick as a jungle, and after a heavy downpour it smells like a tropical rain forest. In the fall, depending on the strength and direction of the wind, the air can smell like salted fish, as it takes on the aroma of an oyster bed that has been exposed by a very low tide. And in the winter (in north Florida we do get a complete change of seasons, however short), trees just stand there in the water, naked, like they just got out of the shower. Well, this is when my nostrils are filled with the smell of wood, particularly cypress and cedar.

Another variable is the smell of salt, which depends on the brackishness of the river at any given time. This is hugely affected by the tidal surges from the ocean at the St. Johns' mouth, the amount of rain we have, and the evaporative effects of the sun. What kind of fish we have off our dock on any given day is directly dependent on the amount of salt in the water. A lot of rain can dilute the river's salinity to the point where it drives the shrimp, crabs, and saltwater fish north, up the river, to get closer to where the St. Johns meets the Atlantic. This is also where the fishing village of Mayport, Florida, is located, along with the Mayport Navy Base, the homeport of several large vessels, including a fully operational 100,000-ton aircraft carrier.

Not much farther north of Mayport is another naval base, near St. Mary's, Georgia, homeport for a multibillion-dollar fleet of nuclear submarines.

What's remarkable is that these two Navy bases closely coordinate their ship and submarine movements to avoid disturbing the breeding grounds of the northern right whale, an area several hundred miles long just off the coast of both bases.

I used to look down and see these whales while piloting a P-3 Orion spy plane off the coast of Florida and Georgia (a plane very similar to the one that had a Chinese fighter jet fly into it, forcing it to land in China). A former flight engineer I used to fly with was one of the twenty-four American hostages the Chinese held for a few weeks prior to their release on April 15, 2001.

I sometimes flew as low as two hundred feet over the water, so seeing these whales wasn't hard at all, although I wasn't always sure it was a right whale, or a whale that wasn't quite right enough.

Severely endangered, the northern right whale population has dwindled to just a few hundred in the entire world. Due to the very slow breeding cycle (three to five years), very lengthy gestational period (I mean, really, we're talking about creating a whale!), and the low number of offspring born at a time (twin births are uncommon, and only seven to fifteen calves are born each year worldwide), the recovery of this unique mammalian species is seriously in doubt. With so few being born each year, there may be a genetic bottleneck that so severely restricts the diversity of their gene pool that the overall species starts to suffer like the interbred royalty of old Europe. Fast-moving warships and submarines running under water at over thirty mph right through their breeding area certainly makes the successful survival of this species even more dubious. Getting hit by a submarine will kill any whale. (I actually cruised one thousand feet below the Mediterranean Sea for a few weeks on the USS *Whale*, one of our nuclear attack submarines.)

In the spirit of sportsmanship and a few federal laws to boot, the Navy and Coast Guard are doing their best to help protect the right whales. They keep ships' logs that specifically detail encounters with the migrating pods of these sixty-foot-long mammals. If they see a whale trapped or drowning in the net or gear of a fishing boat, the boat's captain could get slapped with a huge fine and possible prison sentence if he is proved negligent.

The unusual name, the right whale, came to be for several reasons. First, this particular species of whale was slow moving and easy to kill. Second, relative to other whale species, this whale contained an unusually large amount of oil (used for lubrication and for oil lamps). It also had a lot of baleen, the strange non-teeth in a whale's mouth designed to filter out plankton and shrimp for food. Baleen was used for making corsets, hair brushes, and a variety of other household items.

Last, this particular species of leviathan floated readily on the surface of the ocean after it was killed, unlike most whale species, which quickly sink to the bottom. This made it the "right whale" for whalers to hunt, ultimately earning it that unlucky nickname and helping to make it the most endangered whale in the world.

If only three hundred years ago some farsighted whaler-turned-marine biologist had named it the northern wrong whale! There'd be billions of them by now.

But enough about the right whale, or even the wrong whale. It must be obvious to you by now that I'm a huge fan of whales. I'm fascinated by the world's largest animals. Blue whales exceed in size the largest dinosaurs ever to walk the face of the earth. Whales have been known to swim up the St. Johns River, though I doubt any have swam past our dock. But if I ever see that happen, or anyone else does, for that matter, you can be sure I'll write about it.

Something that has always fascinated me is how dramatically the variety of bird species that we see out on our dock differs from that in our cypress swamp just a few hundred yards away. In the oak and cypress trees of the swamp we see giant barred owls and Cooper's hawks snagging wild mice and lizards from the bushes, ruby-throated hummingbirds with their beaks deep in colorful red swamp flowers, large red-crowned pileated woodpeckers pecking at termites and ants in hollowed-out dead trees, bobwhite quail and wild turkeys kicking up for seed, and a large variety of migrating warblers. Over the water, there are kingfishers diving at swirls of baitfish, bufflehead ducks skimming the brackish water's surface for food, several different kinds of leggy egrets, cranes and wood storks walking the oyster beds spread out among the marsh grass, and the majestic bald eagle cruising the shoreline at high speed, looking for an osprey with a fresh fish that it can steal from its smaller cousin. This habit makes the bald eagle an interesting choice as a symbol of the United States of America . . . maybe a symbol of our entrepreneurial opportunism. If my memory serves me correctly, I think Ben Franklin's choice for our national bird was the wild turkey— but in terms of magnificent physical presence and power, and majesty in flight, I'll take the bald eagle over the wild turkey any day.

As much as I enjoy bird-watching, particularly during the spring and the fall when just about anything could be stopping in for a night of rest in the middle of a migratory flight, I have always been a sucker for mammals. I think it's because baby mammals are guaranteed adorable. Have you ever seen a baby raccoon or rabbit or fox or bear cub that wasn't too cute for words? And what baby mammals lose in cuteness as they mature into adult animals, they gain in the fascinating way in which they learn to adapt to their environment and in the way they develop unique habits and skills in order to survive. I have always been extremely interested in the scientific observation of animal behavior. It has always intrigued me. Behavior of human beings, well, sometimes I can hardly be bothered.

On our nature walk we see rabbits rooting for grass and wildflowers, raccoons digging for clams and crabs, and armadillos digging for ants, termites, and grubs. We see possums and skunks scrounging for anything they can get their paws on. Sometimes we even see gray fox chasing gray squirrels.

(A little-known animal fact is that the gray fox is the only North American canine that can actually climb tall trees. And they do it routinely, not only to get at squirrels and squirrels' nests but to escape predators such as coyotes and wolves, as well as to take midday siestas.)

To walk among God's many unique and reclusive creatures is a privilege I never take for granted. I feel sorry for the people trapped in cities with only rats, mice, pigeons, stray cats and dogs, and other humans to engage with. I see God's hand at work most when I am deep in the woods, among the trees. The diversity of animal life is, to me, God's special touch. God's artistry.

And there's even more of God's artwork down at the dock. We also have otters, mink, and the all-pervasive nutria, which looks like a giant muskrat on steroids. It can grow to almost the size of a beaver, but has a round muskratlike tail instead of the flat tail of a beaver. Nutria were originally imported from South America to be bred for fur, but a couple of them obviously escaped (if you think rabbits and mink have a bad reputation in the rapid-breeding department, nutria make those critters look like part of the church choir). Anyway, gators love nutria—but not for their luxuriant fur coats.

I have always had an extremely strong interest in reptiles, too. Even though I didn't start talking until relatively late, I started reading much earlier than most kids. I was reading fairly comprehensive books on the great reptiles at a rather early age. I knew the names of just about every dinosaur known at the time. My greatest disappointment was that I had been born 200 million years too late to see a dinosaur alive—or to be a dinosaur's meal!

It wasn't long before I came to realize that turtles, snakes, and lizards were the next best thing. Not only that, but they were generally more common and easier to observe in the wild than most other mammals. They were easier to catch as well.

My fascination with reptiles, which began with dinosaurs when I was a child, continues to this day. One of the most pre-historic creatures I observed on our nature walk was a huge female alligator snapper. I watched all one hundred pounds of her lumbering from the river through the mud, laboring to get to higher land. Then I watched her patiently excavate a gallon-sized hole with her hind feet and deposit ninety eggs, which looked like Ping-Pong balls, down into the bottom of it, her eyes tearing, like her larger sea-turtle cousins do when they lay their eggs.

Mission accomplished, she used her back legs to cover the hole with dirt, hopefully well enough that a foraging raccoon or skunk couldn't sniff out the eggs and gobble them up.

People are typically not fans of these big, ugly, and some-what dangerous turtles, and when they happen upon one lay-ing eggs in their backyard, they often blow its head off with a shotgun. Knowing this somewhat strange tradition, I picked this one up by the tail—the only safe way to carry one without having your hand bitten off—carried her down our dock, and dropped her into the water where she could easily swim away. Hopefully, I'll see her when she again emerges from the river next year to lay another clutch of eggs, following her motherly instincts as she has probably been doing for about seventy-five years now, given her enormous size.

Not particularly prehistoric-looking, just plain funny-looking, are giant soft-shelled turtles, one of the more bizarre creatures you're likely ever to see. These large freshwater turtles—as much as thirty inches long—have a long snorkel-like nose and strangely angry-looking humanlike eyes. They also have a very dangerous bite, almost as bad as that of a snapping turtle of equal size. And with their snakelike necks so deceptively long, they can reach out and bite you from much farther away than you would think!

Even though adult snapping turtles and soft-shelled turtles can, if big enough, take off your entire hand, their tiny hatchlings are harmless and unusual pets. Just don't let your kids flush them down the toilet when they get too big, creating another story of a giant mutant turtle or alligator in the sewers. Soft and brown, about the size and flatness of a quarter, baby soft-shelled turtles can live in a tank full of small fish, until they grow to the point where the fish start disappearing at a faster and faster rate. The nicest and smartest thing you can do then, after you have observed them for a while and learned a little something about them, is to release them back into their natural habitat, ideally right where you first found them.

To a lot of southern folk in these parts, both the snapping turtle and the soft-shelled turtle make fine dining. That means better than armadillo, but not as good as possum, and not even close to coon or gator tail. I've tried turtle—tasted like chicken to me. (I wonder what the people in the world who eat a lot of turtle would say to their first taste of chicken—tastes like turtle?)

Turtles generally prefer to live in the water, but there is an exception to this rule: the colorful box turtle. A dark turtle whose shell and skin are splashed with orange and yellow, it's called a "box" turtle because it is the only turtle that can close up its shell like a box as a form of armored protection—especially from marauding raccoons and absentminded people.

I've been a huge fan of box turtles ever since I was five years old, when my father and I and my younger sister Greta discovered one while on a Sunday morning hike in the woods near our home. My dad picked up the turtle, gave it a curious look as it closed up its shell, and then stuck it in his back pocket like a wallet. We continued our hike. When we finally got back home, Dad—who tipped the scales at well over two hundred pounds at the time—had forgotten about the whole turtle encounter, and was about to sit down . . . until Greta and I pleaded with him to give us back our turtle first.

I must have really worried for that turtle, connected with that turtle, even become that turtle for a spell, in a Zen-like way. Maybe that's when my passion and love and ability to empathize with all of God's creatures first began. In the back pocket of my father's khaki trousers.

Box turtles are one of the all-time greatest pets for children to have, as long as you can keep them eating regularly. If you can't get a box turtle to eat in a few days, something is wrong, and you should release it back where you found it. But it should not be hard to get these turtles to eat—they go absolutely nuts over the earthworms you can find in your backyard on a rainy day.

Dr. John Rossi, a herpetologist widely known as The Cold-Blooded Vet because of his extraordinary knowledge of all creatures cold and slimy, believes that earthworms are such a perfectly nutritional food for box turtles (some argue that they're perfect for humans as well) that they can thrive on a diet of earthworms and nothing else, although we've discovered they enjoy fruit, bread, and scrambled eggs, too. The animals in the Goss menagerie eat pretty damn well.

Box turtles are fairly common in our neighborhood, especially after a heavy rain or during their mating season—which to male box turtles seems to be all the time, though the females appear more amiable in spring—and the males are forever out scurrying about in their quest to meet nice lady friends. Peggy and I sometimes find box turtles mating on a woodsy trail we jog on by our home, the male perched very high and awkwardly on top of the female's shell, incredibly balanced, snapping at the back of his lover's neck but never actually biting her. Gets me thinking, but Peggy jogs on.

We've sometimes had four or five box turtles scurrying around our backyard at once. You can always tell which are the males. Their necks stretched high, red eyes bulging, they are always on the prowl, very territorial, masters of their domain . . . kind of like Navy pilots.

In males, the bottom shell, called the plastron, has a very obvious concave indentation, allowing it to neatly fit the top of the female's upper shell, called the carapace, when they mate. Females normally have brown eyes and are generally more reclusive and less likely to be out and about. Their bottom shell is flat to keep them stabilized on the forest floor when they get together for conjugal visits. I mention this only because with most reptiles and amphibians, identifying which is the male and which is the female is not an easy task. It's a snap to tell a female box turtle from a male—she's the one sitting on the back of the motorcycle.

We've had a pet box turtle living in our home for years now, but I'll share more with you about Rocky's close buddy Little Rascal later.

Box turtles generally prefer land, but they can and do spend a great deal of time in and around water. A tortoise, however, is a dedicated land dweller, definitely preferring to be dry rather than wet. Often, tortoises don't drink water even when given the opportunity, but instead extract all their moisture from the fresh grasses and wildflowers that they eat. Big brown Florida gopher tortoises are somewhat common in our area, but they are listed as an endangered species nationwide, and you'll pay a large fine if you're caught messing with one of the forty foot-long burrows they dig in sandy areas.

Gopher-tortoise burrows are also home to a great variety of other animals indigenous to Florida, including six-foot-long diamondback rattlesnakes and the eastern indigo snake—a very shiny thick black snake with a red chin—that grows to over nine feet long, making it the longest snake native to North America. Very friendly to humans, the indigo loves to snack on the cottonmouth water moccasin; the handsome indigo snake is apparently immune to the moccasin's venom.

We have a big Texas indigo snake named Tex as a pet. He's as friendly as a dog and eats just about anything I throw in his cage. He's a thick six-footer, and holding such an impressive and utterly fascinating creature in my hands is always a thrill. I'll get back to Tex later, but I can tell you that fear of snakes is *not* innate among humans.

When we are very young we have a natural and innate fear of only two things: heights and loud noises. All of our other fears are learned, typically from our parents during our early years. I believe most fears can be conquered through greater understanding, and through the years I have helped many people get over their fear of reptiles and amphibians, particularly snakes, which are among the world's most fascinating creatures.

Many people think snakes are slimy. They are not. They are dry and smooth and very nice to the touch. When I get people who are afraid of snakes to hold one of our pet ones, this is one of the first things they say, and their fear of snakes normally melts away in just moments. If all our fears could be put to rest through greater understanding as easily as this, a lot of prejudices and phobias would be gone for good and the world would be a better place because of it. By helping to educate people out of being fearful of snakes, or flying, or cancer, I hope in some small way to make the world a better place.

But let's get back to nature, especially to our nature walk and our dock on the St. Johns River.

A world-famous fishing spot, the St. Johns River, I've heard, is the only northerly flowing river in the United States, but because I haven't floated all of them yet, please don't quote me on that.

Because of its proximity to the Atlantic Ocean and because salinity varies from day to day depending on the rain and tides, this giant river contains just about every imaginable variety of fresh- and saltwater fish. This includes largemouth bass, massive tarpon, stingrays, eels, ten-foot-long sturgeon, speckled sea trout, redfish, enormous carp, flounder, sunfish and crappies, huge catfish, blue crabs, shrimp, mullet—loads of mullet. The mullet keep things interesting when we are on our dock because they are always jumping high out of the water to give us a good look at their infamous mullet faces. Sometimes, mullet actually jump out of the water and land on the dock right next to us.

And without a doubt there are sharks in the river, especially where it joins the Atlantic. We once found a 250-pound, eight-foot-long tarpon, dead, next to our dock. The scales on this creature were the size of playing cards—enormous. It had a huge bite out of it, about a foot behind its head. Almost definitely from a shark.

It seems every couple of years, Florida has a sudden summertime rash of shark attacks, usually from bull or black-tip sharks, which don't have a clue they're attacking a human and not some food thrashing about in the water. I read about a boy who had lost his arm to a bull shark. His uncle ran into the water, dragged out the shark, killed it, cut open its stomach, and removed the boy's arm from it. The boy was rushed to the hospital where a team of neurosurgeons reattached his arm. Talk about a miracle!

Since records started being kept in Florida, there have been 438 confirmed shark attacks and only 21—less than 5 percent—were fatal. Australia has had 323 confirmed attacks, but 152—almost 50 percent—were fatal. That's because in Australia, its not a little six-foot black-tip or bull shark grabbing hold of you, it's a sixteen-foot great white, as in *Jaws.*

When I was the assistant navigator of the nuclear aircraft carrier USS *Carl Vinson,* I saw great whites on the Pacific Ocean's surface looking for prey as we steamed past the Farallon Islands on our way to Pearl Harbor. The great whites of the Farallon Islands are famous for their seal-tossing maneuver. *National Geographic* did a remarkable television special about this unique form of hunting and playing. When a 20-foot, 4,000-pound great white grabs hold of a 500-pound seal, that seal sometimes gets tossed like a beach ball high into the air. If a seal ever ended up on the flight deck, about forty feet above the ocean's surface, from my unique viewpoint even higher up on the ship's navigation bridge with the captain, I'd be the first to know. And I'm sure one of these days its going to happen, if it hasn't happened already.

Sharks, whales, and dolphins have always fascinated me for their unpredictable nature, their size, and their intelligence, in that order. Bottle-nosed dolphins, like whales, have been known to swim up our river, but I haven't seen one go by our dock yet. However, I've spent a lot of time with dolphins on several different occasions in my life. While boating with my parents near Siesta Key, Florida, while doing catch-and-release fishing for sailfish and marlin in Guatemala with my brother and friends, and especially while navigating a huge nuclear aircraft carrier for months on end across the Pacific Ocean, dolphins have been there, like angels of the sea, joyfully leaping out of the water just off the bow, guiding the way.

As a boy growing up in the Northeast, the television show *Flipper* entertained me endlessly, and I was envious beyond belief that a kid could live in Florida, on the water, and have so many wild animals as pets, especially a pet dolphin that appeared to be about ten times smarter than the kid's park-ranger dad.

Of course, Peggy and I and the twins love seeing the dolphins when we visit an aquarium, but having the St. Johns River at the end of our dock is almost like having a world-class aquarium just a stone's skip away.

The water's edge is the ideal place for observing all forms of flora and fauna. It is also the perfect place to reflect not only on nature but on the very nature of life itself. I love the water. But I love the water's edge even more. That is where life truly abounds.

Occasionally, while sitting at the end of our dock, a big gray head will pop out of the water at my feet. This head, the size of a large watermelon, will look at me with its whiskered muzzle and small eyes and then let out a very loud snort of air, like someone blowing his nose. If this creature is as startled by me as I am by it, it will crest its two-thousand-pound body out of the water and make an enormous splash, showering me with water and creating a shock wave that actually shakes our dock.

The visitor, of course, is the endangered Florida manatee, of which there are only approximately a few thousand still alive in the world. Thankfully, many of them seem to like staying all year long in our part of the St. Johns River. Unfortunately, some of the manatees we see have giant gouges in their backs and fins where they were nicked by the propellers of speed-boats. The slow-moving manatees are unable to maneuver fast enough to avoid these horrendous injuries.

Strict speed limits now govern the waters where manatees are commonly seen. And there are some even tougher penalties to pay if the Fish and Game Department catches you breaking those limits. Nonetheless, many manatees are hurt or killed this way each year.

The injured manatees inspired me in a way. If they could tolerate and survive chunks of their bodies being haphazardly removed by wild speedboaters, then surely I could tolerate the removal of a section of my ear by a skilled surgeon.

Sometimes Peggy, the twins, and I would quietly swim beside the manatees using snorkeling equipment, especially in Crystal River, a favorite place of ours. It's a freshwater river that feeds into the Gulf of Mexico, and it's only a few hours' drive south of us. The best part of the river is the gorgeous springs, where millions of gallons of crystal clear, 72-degree water bubbles up from the super-deep Florida aquifer. In the dead of winter, even Florida's waters can get rather chilly, but not here.

Around Christmas, the warm waters of Crystal Springs sometimes attract hundreds of manatees into an area of only about an acre or two. The Parks and Wildlife rangers rope off the area, but people are permitted to swim just outside the enclosure, where there are still many manatees to be seen, especially mama manatees—cows—nursing their two-hundred-pound calves.

Although you are not permitted to swim after them, you are allowed to stroke and pet the manatees who approach you. Unbelievably, this happens all the time. The manatees, even the babies, seem to love having their chins scratched and their bellies rubbed. And nothing is cuter than a baby manatee rolling over on your lap, looking deeply into your eyes and begging you for a good belly rub.

I guess I am so fond of manatees because they are so large and yet so gentle. With their immense size, they could really throw their weight around if they wanted to, but instead they choose to be incredibly sweet and graceful. When they stick their seaweed-covered heads out of the water they sometimes look like mermaids—really, really ugly mermaids, but mermaids nonetheless.

Besides manatees, there are alligators in the St. Johns River, some of them very large—as long as sixteen feet, if you believe the photographs, skulls, and gator skins at Whitey's Fish Camp, the local fish restaurant up the river from our home. From our dock I have seen only teenagers, mere five- or six-footers, their ten-inch-long heads protruding from the water for a minute or two, only to sink beneath the surface for another few moments, before their heads come up ten or twenty yards away for another breath of air. I'm still keeping my eye out for monster granddaddy alligators, but they're generally wise enough to forage and feed under the cover of darkness. That's how they end up getting so big: It's harder for poachers to find them late at night.

But the potential for big gators hasn't kept us off our dock at night. Excruciatingly early one morning, son Brian shook me awake. He had a sleeping bag under each arm. Eyes heavy, we walked down to the end of our dock, spread out our bags, and lay flat on our backs to watch a meteor shower that we had read about the day before in the *Florida Times-Union*.

Now, I had gotten up early for a lot of highly heralded meteor showers over the past thirty or so years, and none of them had been worth the effort. Yet I couldn't bear to tell that to Brian. So, since he had made the effort, as the dad, I would have to make the effort, too.

But let me tell you something—this meteor shower was worth the effort. It was *spectacular*. Over the course of the next three hours, Brian and I (Peggy and Christie joined us later) saw hundreds and then thousands of meteors streaking overhead, from horizon to horizon across the four-mile expanse of the St. Johns River. And although not one meteor was even remotely as immense as the one I spotted in my backyard soon after I was diagnosed with cancer, to see countless meteors streaking across the heavens at the exact same moment in time and space—well that is a *very* impressive aerial display, well worth getting out of bed to see, even at 3:00 A.M.

The property our house sits on is special in its own right. When I was just a small child, I had a recurring dream about catching fish and other small creatures in an imaginary stream or pond I visualized flowing through the backyard of my boyhood home in New Jersey. I remember other boys my age, Greg O'Neil being one of them, saying they'd had a similar dream. Maybe it is some kind of child-to-adolescent rite of passage dream—though I sometimes still have that same dream, thirty-five years later.

When Peg and I and the kids were transferred to Florida more than twelve years ago, after I had served a tour of duty on the giant nuclear aircraft carrier USS *Carl Vinson*, I immediately fell in love with the house Peggy had scouted out. A beautiful home, yes, but the kicker was that a tiny stream actually did flow through the backyard, exactly the way I had dreamed. After we bought the house, I set to work completing that dream. Working around a six-month deployment to Iceland to spy on Russian submarines, I built a pond big enough to hold some largemouth bass—really big largemouth bass—loads of sunfish, a five-pound catfish, plus a half-dozen turtles (red-eared sliders, to be exact—the grown-up version of the tiny green water turtles we used to buy in dime stores before they were outlawed years ago due to a salmonella scare), bullfrogs, some small water snakes—even a baby alligator. But I'll get to him in just a moment (the tip of my finger *still* hurts when I think about him).

The pond we built turned out beautifully and now serves as a favored swimming hole for Christie and Brian and their friends. A lot of the families in our neighborhood have swimming pools, but this—this is different. It is *loaded* with critters of every shape and size. The largemouth bass that Brian put into the pond after catching it in the river has really grown up. Nicknamed Big Mouth Billy the Bass, he now eats whole uncooked hotdogs and hamburgers, sometimes right out of our hands, on a regular basis. If you don't think largemouth bass are aggressive, well, you just haven't seen Big Mouth Billy in action. He might have even eaten a baby alligator that used to be in our pond.

Now, I didn't plan on having an alligator living in our backyard. But one day an acquaintance of mine rescued a baby gator from getting run over by a car.

I learned a lot about crocodilians the day he came over with that baby alligator in his hand. It was tiny—must have been only a few weeks old, about seven inches long and only a few ounces in weight. It must have just hatched from one of the several dozen eggs its mother had laid in the three-foot-high grass nest she had created. Grass nests have a dual purpose: first, to incubate the eggs through the heat of decomposition, and second, to keep the eggs hidden from predators such as raccoons, water moccasins, kingsnakes, and indigo snakes, which love gator eggs almost as much as they love baby gators.

There is an old wives' tale that an alligator has almost no muscular strength to open its jaws, but has a tremendous, almost supernatural strength to close them. I am here to tell you from personal experience that's no old wives' tale. It's true.

Here's how I know. My friend handed me the newly hatched gator to look at and asked if he could release it in our backyard pond. "Sure," I said, knowing that watching a baby gator grow up in our pond would be a whole lot of fun, especially after he got bigger. I held the little gator in my left hand and gently stroked his snout with my right hand as he grunted excitedly at me. The velociraptor scene in the movie *Jurassic Park* should have been ample warning, but it wasn't. I mean, it appeared so harmless and friendly before it attacked. The next thing I knew, that little gator had the tip of my right index finger halfway down his throat.

The thing that was most amazing to me was not the sharpness of those teeth, which were plenty sharp, don't get me wrong. Instead, it was the incredible pressure that tiny set of jaws had upon my finger. It was excruciating—I felt like my finger was being crushed. It made me want to rip that baby gator off my hand even if a large piece of my finger went with it. Instead, I waited patiently for him to tire of my finger taste. When he finally did, he was gently placed in the pond. I haven't seen him since. But I have a feeling that either Big Mouth Billy the Bass or a hungry raccoon has.

Getting bitten by that baby gator and by countless other wild and domestic animals over the course of my life hasn't made me love animals any less. In fact, the sometimes painful physical contact I've had with Mother Nature through the years hasn't taken any toll on me. Rather, it has been rejuvenating. I believe with absolute certainty that when we are in extremis, connecting with animals and with nature itself is the key to our finding ourselves and the inner strengths that get us through the great challenges that may lie before us.

After decades of studies, researchers who specialize in the preferences and effects of nature on our moods and the human spirit came to some interesting conclusions. One of the more compelling is that people are most captivated and inspired by "mystery" landscapes—those settings that invite our curiosity by having a hidden bend in a footpath or a clump of trees or bushes obscuring another feature. Intrigue and exploration of the unknown in nature help to pump us up in ways that are healthy for both our bodies and our minds, while boredom, routine, and familiarity have a destructive effect on us.

It's also been demonstrated that bringing animals into nursing homes and other caregiving institutions to permit residents to see and hold dogs, cats, ferrets, even turtles and snakes, creates a stimulation that is both exciting and calming for them, often helping even those with severely impaired mental and motor functions.

Bird-watchers report that when they spot a rare species during a walk in the woods, they feel the same endorphin "high" as long-distance runners achieve.

Even more to the point, taking in all this nature, right there in my own backyard, was—and still is—a tremendous boost to my human spirit. It was actually a form of supercharging, if I may be so bold as to describe the human spirit in the mechanical terms of combining fuel, air, and fire under far greater than normal pressure to extract far greater than normal performance.

I believe now, more than ever, that a boost to the human

spirit provides a direct boost to the immune system. And cancer is, almost by definition, a disease of a failing immune system; first, at a local level, and then, at a systemic level, spreading like a completely out-of-control fire throughout the internal systems of the body.

And the single best way to fight an illness—in particular, a disease like cancer—is to arm yourself with a supercharged immune system. It does not guarantee you 100 percent remission from disease 100 percent of the time. But an attitude like this, in which you consciously put yourself in places and environments that are good for you and that help you to reaffirm your basic desire and will to live, will always help you get the most out of your remaining time on earth, with your family and friends and all the other physical as well as spiritual things in life you have come to love and value so dearly.

What's the value you put on your life or the life of your loved ones? If you truly realized that value, would you continue living life in the rat race? Or would you choose to spend more quality time enjoying private moments with your family and closest friends at a quiet lake, with your cell phone turned off?

Besides my family and friends, one way that I tapped in to my love of nature and of all animals in a very large and meaningful way was simply by spending more time at the water's edge on our dock, our nature walk, and our pond and waterfall. You might say, "Well, we don't have a pond or a waterfall in our backyard." That's the point. Neither did we. So we saved our money and we busted our butts and we dug a pond, and built a waterfall, nature walk, and dock. You don't always have to go to nature. You can bring nature to you.

There are countless other ways to tap in to the healing power of nature, some as simple as taking a walk in your local park and feeding the squirrels or pigeons a little something from your lunch, if that's all you can do at the moment. But I hope you will seek out more than that. If you really get involved and fall in love with the great outdoors and all its denizens, it will be the best thing in the world for you.

I still had plenty of homework to do on this subject because I knew, I could feel it deep down in my bones, that the closer I got to my surgery, the more I would need every bit of healing power available.

4

Bad Time to Be a Rodent

*T*hings were bad. So far, I'd been diagnosed with cancer and received a second opinion which was far worse than the first. It reminded me of the old joke about the doctor who gives his patient some bad news. "I want a second opinion," complains the patient. The doctor obliges. "Okay, you're ugly too!"

After the second opinion at Shands and then a third opinion from the Armed Forces Institute of Pathology in Bethesda, Maryland, I had to accept that I had a very deadly form of cancer. It was time to face the music.

I wanted two things. One, to learn as much about cancer and cancer survival as fast as was humanly possible. And two, to be operated on without any more delays. I kept going back to the basic premise I had learned about highly malignant cancers like melanoma: Every second that goes by provides the tumor with an opportunity to spread, drastically altering the battle in favor of the enemy. I wanted the cutting to get started and get started *now*. I badgered my doctors for the earliest possible surgery date. A few days after my second CAT scan, and armed with a confirming report from the Armed Forces Institute of Pathology, I was scheduled for an entire day of surgery—show time at seven in the morning. Tomorrow morning. That didn't give me a lot of time to think about it and I was glad about that. There was still a whole lot more I had to learn, but I knew that delaying the surgery any longer would be a huge mistake.

I had spent one of my last two-eared days studying articles in *The Journal of the American Medical Association* and *The New England Journal of Medicine*. One particular article on malignant melanoma really caught my interest. It was on the effects that a substance called DHEA had on laboratory mice that had been medically induced to develop deadly malignant melanoma tumors (definitely a bad time to be a rodent).

This article made me laugh out loud because it reminded me of a rather amusing statement that made light of the whole question as to what caused cancer. Was it tobacco, the sun, alcohol, our drinking water supply, asbestos, low fiber, white bread, sugar, air pollution, sugar-free soda, hot dogs— we have all seen the huge list of foods and substances that have been labeled as carcinogenic. So when I read that "It's recently been discovered that medical research causes cancer in mice" and then read this research paper on DHEA, I had to laugh at the irony of it all, because suddenly, in its own strange way, directly related to my life, even this joke was no longer really a joke.

Since there were not that many research papers available on melanoma (and virtually none on amelanotic melanoma) I turned my focus on this particular article and read it thoroughly.

As I said, by this time I was fairly well studied up on malignant melanoma, but the subject of DHEA was brand new to me.

Some cancer researchers took a large group of young, genetically similar laboratory mice that were all the same age and split them into three equal groups. The researchers then injected fast-growing malignant melanoma tumors under the skin of two of the three groups. In a matter of months the injected mice developed observable tumors. Equally observable, as the weeks and months continued, their hair turned gray, their coats grew coarser and thinner, muscle-to-body-fat ratios shifted—and their tumors grew larger.

At a certain point in time, the researchers started giving large daily doses of DHEA to half of the cancerous mice. Remarkably, the mice given the DHEA began to show a significant slowing in tumor growth and in some cases even reduction in tumor size, compared to the cancerous mice that had not received the DHEA.

At the same time, the cancerous, non-DHEA supplemented mice began to die off at the rate you would expect any animal whose body had begun to manifest the ravages of cancer.

Then there were the mice in the control group. They had not been given cancer *or* DHEA. They were aging normally (lab mice have a normal life span of about twenty-four months) and were developing graying hair, thinning and coarser coats, higher fat-to-muscle ratios with tendencies toward obesity, and they demonstrated signs of reduced vitality and energy levels—reduced climbing and exploring, reduced interest in sexual activity—their own, that is . . . all typical signs of aging in mice.

Now here's the fascinating part. The mice that were given both the cancer and the DHEA had smoother, thicker coats of hair, more muscle and less body fat, and had greater demonstrated energy levels and vitality than even the noncancerous mice of the same age.

In other words, the daily DHEA supplements were not only causing the melanoma tumors to shrink and in some cases to disappear, they were also causing the mice to look, act, and feel younger, both inside and out, than the control mice.

The researchers were stunned by the implications of this—and so was I. But as I started to research and learn more about DHEA, its effects on the human body and on the bodies of other animals no longer seemed very surprising.

DHEA (short for dehydroepiandrosterone) is a hormone naturally produced by our adrenal glands. As one of the predominant hormones in the human body, it has a very interesting life cycle in both men and women. When we are babies, our adrenal glands produce very small amounts of DHEA. At age ten, our production of this hormone starts to ramp up. By age twenty (when so many of us feel immortal) it is the most actively produced hormone in our bodies and is the most highly measurable hormone in our blood, earning it the nickname "the master control hormone" by some researchers in endocrinology. These scientists are struck by the gentle yet very significant effect DHEA appears to have on the production of the other vitally important components in the hormonal stew we call the human body, major hormones such as testosterone, androgen, estrogen, insulin, adrenaline and a host of others.

As we pass our twentieth year, DHEA production starts to drop off—slowly at first—in a way quite different from that of other hormones. For instance, at age thirty, our DHEA production is about half what it was when we were twenty. At age forty, it is half of what it was when we were thirty, and so forth. This exponentially accelerating decline continues until we reach age seventy, when the typical man or woman is no longer producing a biologically significant amount of this hormone.

What happens to most people when they reach their seventies and beyond? Unfortunately, at the end of the typical human life cycle, we suddenly start to age very dramatically, get extremely frail, get sick, and then die.

The researchers concluded that DHEA was strengthening the mice's immune systems and allowing them to fight the melanoma. I thought this was an extremely significant discovery—not only to me, but to the entire human race. Because although most people don't have to deal with malignant melanoma, a lot of us have to deal with other forms of cancer and *all* of us have to deal with the effects of aging.

If raising our blood levels of DHEA back to their more youthful levels really has such a dramatic effect on our general wellness, that could be something huge for mankind over the long term, I figured. And very huge over the very short term for me.

What if? Well, the medical journal what-if'd me—and that's all I needed to hear. I love being what-if'd. Being what-if'd raises the possibilities that you are going to learn something new—and that doesn't happen every day.

I went on to research the possible side effects of DHEA

and found no known risks for low-dose supplementation except one—it might cause overstimulation of the male prostate gland, increasing a man's chance of getting prostate cancer over the long term. Prostate cancer is another terrible disease, but my concern at this time was effectively fighting malignant melanoma over the short term. And, thankfully, certain studies have since disproved the potential link of DHEA to prostate cancer.

Inexpensive and easy to find in just about any food or drugstore today, DHEA was a lot harder to find when I was first diagnosed with cancer. But find it I did, and just before my surgery I started taking a 100 mg tablet every morning. My doctors didn't care if I took DHEA or not—I think they thought it might have a positive placebo effect on me. And maybe it did. But, between you and me, I believe it did a whole lot more. Some of my friends, upon learning I was taking DHEA, started taking it also. But I insisted they first do their homework on it, like I had done mine.

That's not the only mouse research I found interesting. Another study, this one by Dr. Jaak Panksepp, a neuroscientist at Bowling Green State University, discovered that rodents responded to certain unusual stimuli (tickling on the tummy, for instance) by, believe it or not, laughing. "It's more like a chirp," said Panksepp, who feels these findings could help other scientists learn more about the brain systems that help to elevate the mood and regulate happiness, something DHEA is also supposed to do.

I wash down my morning DHEA tablet with water. Oceans of it. You see, another thing I discovered through my studies was that I was not drinking nearly enough water each day to maintain a powerful immune system response 24/7. I'm definitely not talking about expensive bottled water, just regular old tap water, which in the United States is 99 percent cleaner and more pure than all the rest of the world's drinking water supplies put together. Large quantities of clear fresh water are vital for flushing the toxins from our blood via our kidney's filtering system and its production of urine.

Our bodies evolved to conserve water, in case of a drought. So our kidneys are designed to preserve our internal body fluids for us, which is mostly water, in preparation for that inevitable dry spell, *except* when they sense that we are drinking more than enough water, even for a long dry spell. Then the kidneys will stabilize in a more hydrated state.

You must drink regular clear water if you want to help your body. It can't be any liquid you want, and especially not beverages containing caffeine or alcohol. Why? Because caffeine and alcohol are very powerful chemical dehydrants, causing you to lose more fluid than you take in, wringing out vital water from your circulatory system and the 65 trillion living cells within your body, forcing your kidneys into a cycle that reduces the essential filtering and purifying of your blood that they were designed to do. So if you enjoy a cup of coffee in the morning, a glass of iced tea at lunch, and maybe a glass of wine at night, it's okay, just as long as you force yourself to overcompensate by consuming significant quantities of water every day, especially in the morning when you wake up.

The expert on this subject, and the man who personally educated me on the chronic dehydration that many of us suffer from, is my friend Dr. Batmanghelidj. A brilliant M.D. once sentenced to die in an Iranian prison, he's the author of the remarkable book *Your Body's Many Cries for Water*. In it, he describes a variety of medical symptoms many adults and children experience due to chronic dehydration. Some are directly related to having a reduced immune response, never good in the case of cancer and so many other diseases.

What happens to that glass of water you just drank? It moves quickly—faster than you would expect it to, and much faster than, say, a steak sandwich—from the stomach into the small intestine, where it is very rapidly absorbed directly into our blood by the millions of tiny capillaries that surround this organ. By drinking lots of water, we are diluting, cleansing, and, in many ways, improving our blood chemistry. This is very important. Maintaining adequate levels of hydration with water is one of the most important ways we can simply and inexpensively solve many heart, blood, and circulatory problems.

Many doctors now believe that we are—essentially—our blood chemistry. Why? Blood, being pumped nonstop by the heart, supplies water, oxygen, hormones, and nutrition to every one of the estimated 65 trillion living cells that make up the human body. One drop of our blood contains about 250 million red, white, and platelet blood cells floating in a sea of plasma. Over 90 percent of our blood is water. Ipso facto, if we don't have a lot of water in our bodies, we don't have a lot of blood in our bodies. And I tend to think that having a lot of blood inside me is a good thing, especially in the event of an emergency. Bleeding is good. When you stop bleeding—when you run out of blood—now that's bad. The water we drink dilutes the toxins in our blood. And it's that same water that serves as the soluble solution to transport these toxins out of our bodies and into the sewers, where they belong.

I've got to tell you, I'm awfully glad that this is all handled automatically for us and we don't have to supervise each event that happens in our bodies. But we do have to supervise what goes in and out of our mouths, noses, eyes, ears, etc. Our blood chemistry is very connected to the concentration or dilution of our red blood cells, which is significantly a function of our daily water intake.

I saw the light after reading Dr. Batmanghelidj's book. Now I tank up every morning like a camel getting ready to cross the desert. While taking a shower after my morning workout, I open my mouth and drink as much water from the shower faucet as my stomach can possibly hold. Water assimilates into our blood much faster than solid food. All that water is in my blood in less than an hour, raising my blood volume dramatically. With that rise in blood volume, my kidneys automatically go into a more thorough filtering and cleansing of toxins in my blood. A large glass of water is one of our most remarkable medicines. DHEA is cheap, but tap water is virtually free and available almost everywhere.

But better yet is air. Air is completely free. And getting more air into your lungs and then into your blood through daily activity and aerobic exercise is another tremendous way to supercharge your immune system and enhance your health and your sense of well-being. Besides, it stimulates the release of endorphins, those funky little hormones known for providing the long-distance runner with that "high" that is so much more fulfilling and beneficial for both our bodies and souls than the high that comes from the abuse of drugs and alcohol.

Here are a couple of interesting facts that I learned about our lungs' all-important role in getting oxygen to our red blood cells. Did you know that the redder your blood is, the more oxygen it contains? Blood without oxygen is a very dark purple. Inside each one of our lungs are 300 million little air sacs called alveoli. Each one of these little guys is begging for you to suck in a fresh new oxygen molecule for it to call its own for just a couple of seconds, before it deposits it inside a red blood cell that has stopped by to say hello.

Each red blood cell stoically—maybe even heroically—circulates nonstop throughout our hearts and lungs, picking up and delivering oxygen to all of our bodies' other cells, from the tips of our toes and fingers to the tops of our heads. Amazingly, our entire blood supply washes through our lungs about once a minute. This occurs around 300,000 times to each of our red blood cells before they finally wear out and die, which gives each individual red blood cell about 120 days here on earth. Talk about living an unselfish lifestyle! Thankfully, our bone marrow is constantly producing 3 million of these little heroes per second, to make up for the 3 million red blood cells that are dying inside you per second. It's the liver's job to filter out and get rid of all these dead red blood cells, now no longer bright red but instead a dark brown, by depositing them into the intestines to mix with everything in there on its way to its final destination.

What a change of heart occurs when you are diagnosed with cancer. Suddenly, it's easy to start doing healthier things and things that are better for you, your family, and your friends. I incorporated many changes in my daily routine as I started to prepare for cancer surgery. None of these things is expensive or hard to do.

For instance, not only do I now take a multiple vitamin with minerals every day, but I also, every morning, mix together a weird concoction to put on my cereal. My kids call it "Dad's colon blow." Cute, huh? It is great for preventing colon cancer and it's great for the brain and possibly even the immune system (which is powerfully affected by the brain).

First I get some lecithin soy granules, which are loaded with acetylcholine, a substance that assists in faster and more efficient brain-cell firings between each synapse or brain-cell connection. There are around 100 trillion of these synapses in the average-size brain. That's a big number, 100 trillion. Because I didn't trust I had an average-size brain, I started taking lecithin for maintenance, and maybe even for the improvement of both my cognitive skills and my memory.

I mix the lecithin soy granules with a natural, soluble, high-roughage food called psyllium fiber (it comes from ground-up wheat husks) and mix it in with my cereal. You can imagine . . . anyone who eats something as prosimian as this is guaranteed a cleaned-out exhaust pipe by nine each morning. But seriously, I learned that this combo of lecithin granules and psyllium fiber is vitally important—at least to me—to prevent cancer of the colon; it is also a cheap and easy way to shed excess weight. A high-fiber diet not only soaks up a lot of dietary fats and cholesterol, it speeds what you ate last night through your system so fast that your small intestine doesn't have much of a chance to absorb it. This is especially true regarding the more toxic stuff that's created when it ferments and putrefies in your small intestine and remains there for more than twenty-four hours (a near impossibility if you have a lot of psyllium fiber on your cereal each morning).

Being that I'm only ten pounds over the 185 pounds at which I played middle linebacker for my high school football team and just a few pounds more than my fighting weight when I was a light-heavyweight Golden Gloves boxer twenty-five years ago, it appears my morning cereal concoction is working. It must be, because I've heard Peggy comment to our friends—with some disdain in her voice, I might add— that "I just don't understand it. Bill eats like a pig. He should be three hundred pounds by now."

And finally, there's garlic. It's been discovered that this tasty herb has a powerful immune-boosting property due to the presence of a chemical substance known as allicin; at least that is what researchers at the University of California have said. So maybe it wasn't the smell of the stuff that was keeping vampires away from Transylvania's virgins after all. Maybe it was the allicin.

After learning about the immune-boosting power of the allicin that exists naturally in garlic, I started taking an odor-free enteric-coated garlic tablet with dinner every night. Enteric-coated tablets are specially designed to remain whole and undigested until passing out of your stomach and into your small intestine, dramatically reducing the stomach distress, bad breath, and heartburn associated with mega-dosing yourself with fresh garlic. Enteric-coated garlic tablets are also cheap and available at most food and drugstores. I'm convinced that garlic is good medicine, as good for our bodies as Italian food is good for our souls.

And of course, I think exercise is very important—it seems to help put so many health-related things together in so many different ways: the lungs and the increased air-blood exchange, the faster blood flow through the body and to the extremities, the smoother and more complete digestive/intestinal/urinary tract functioning. Peggy and I try to get a combination walk-run in every morning after the kids have headed off to meet their school bus. There is a wooded dirt road near us that is our preferred exercise route. Since we live in Florida, things really heat up fast, but because this little road is so narrow and it's not paved, it stays much cooler than the other roads in our neighborhood.

Peanut, our Yorkshire terrier, loves to come along with us to chase the many gray squirrels we see each morning. Because Peanut runs more slowly the closer she gets to the squirrels, it seems more like a game for her than actual pursuit. Even the squirrels enjoy it, with the same squirrels waiting by the same trees for her each morning. With the thousands of squirrel encounters Peanut has now had, what is remarkable is that she has yet to actually contact even one squirrel. Except, of course, for the mornings when she touches noses with Rock the Flying Squirrel. She doesn't seem to have a clue that little Rocky is a member of the squirrel family, and he doesn't seem to know that little bit of information either. Rocky thinks he's as human as you or I.

After Peggy and I finish our walk-run, I do ten minutes of flexibility training, followed by a ten-minute chest-and-arm workout, followed by a ten-minute abdominal routine. Then I'm done for the day in regards to aerobic, flexibility, and strength exercise, unless I find the time to get in a little swimming off our dock on the St. Johns River or at a local swim club. But one thing's for certain: I always stay on the move, I always stay active, not only because I like to, but because I know it's good for my body and soul.

But enough about Bill Goss's seven cheap and easy ways to better happiness and health.

Because, in regard to my particular cancer challenge, without a doubt the *most* important thing that needed to happen was this: I got slapped onto a table, knocked out with horse tranquilizer or whatever they use, and a skilled surgeon cut out all of my cancer—and cut it out quick.

So, at the hospital early one morning with Peg at my side, I took off my clothes and changed into a green, loose-fitting hospital gown with my bare-naked butt hanging out the back of it. I then climbed up onto a gurney and some nurses rolled me into a little white area just outside the operating room. I remember my nose filling with the sterile smell of rubbing alcohol. Peggy and I kissed. She wished me luck. Then an anesthesiologist gently stuck a needle into my arm and asked me to start counting backward from ten to zero as I was wheeled into the operating room.

As I reached the number eight, I suddenly felt a chilling rush in my veins. My eyes fell closed.

5

Rocky Becomes My Copilot

I remember opening my eyes and looking up at a very blurred, greenish white world, then suddenly feeling sick to my stomach. I started to gag, but something huge and metallic and monstrous was buried deep down in my throat. I gagged again. I will never quite forget the feeling—kind of like I had been shish-ke-babbed through the mouth. It was awful. I remember Peggy saying to a nearby nurse, "Excuse me, he's waking up—he's trying to talk. Can you get that thing out of his mouth?"

A doctor and a nurse worked for what seemed like an eternity, struggling to extrude this hellish thing from my mouth. Suddenly, *pop*—out shot this shiny-looking device. It looked like a new trowel from the garden department at Wal-Mart. At least that's what it looked like to me from my drugged-out, flat-on-my-back perspective. Later I learned that the nasty thing had a name: endotracheal tube. I hope I never have to eat one of those things for breakfast again.

The pain I started to feel all over my face and head was amazingly intense, as was the terrible nausea, caused by my having been under anesthesia for such an extended length of time. The nausea I had been warned about. But the severity of the pain—that was unexpected. And yet, rather than be dismayed, I welcomed it. Why? Because the pain was the purest and truest and most absolute sign imaginable to me that I had taken the first step to survive cancer. I knew that without pain, I could not have my tumor removed. To have thought that my tumor would go away on its own accord would have been sheer fantasy, and, at the time, neither chemotherapy nor radiation had proven to have any measure of success at curing malignant melanoma. So in my case, pain—pain from major surgery—was a requirement. Pain was good, because it meant I had taken the first—and the most important—step toward becoming healthy again.

Having Peggy right there at my side when I woke up in the recovery room was very important to me. I was so nauseated and disoriented during the first few hours that I am not quite sure what I would have done if she hadn't been there to reassure me that the operation was over and that it was now time to start the healing process.

Brian and Christie did not come to the hospital with Peggy. They were only six years old and Peggy wisely felt that the biology of cell mutations and the history of cancer was a bit over their heads. So she asked them to remember how, when they felt sick, it seemed like they were never going to get better, but they always did. And that this was exactly what was going to happen to Daddy—it would seem like he wasn't going to get better, but that, just like them, he would get better too. Peggy never seemed to give the appearance that the odds were stacked way against me. She was just what the doctor ordered, because if she had lost faith, I might have lost faith.

In many ways, I followed Peggy's lead, because when it comes to saying things to people (even our own children) in a nice and dignified way, Peggy is the best there is. Sometimes I tend to be too blunt . . . not sensitive enough. Maybe it's a guy thing. But I've certainly learned a lot from Peggy through the years in this regard and am a better father and friend because of it.

So I followed Peggy's example in talking with the twins about the cancer challenge we were going through. Honest and direct communication, but simple and full of hope and humor. Our plan was for them to see me after I got home from the hospital, and only then. Peggy was concerned that if Christie and Brian saw me looking all messed up in the hospital and then I didn't go home with them afterward, it would cause them a lot of worry. But if, after three or four days in the hospital, I was able to clean myself up a little, go home, and ask them to help take care of me, well, then my surgery could possibly be turned into a family activity that involved sharing, learning, and maybe even a little bit of fun for Brian and Christie. I'd be able to pretend I was a great big playful monster for them.

One of the first things I did upon regaining consciousness was try to sit up. This was a mistake. As the nurses transferred me from the gurney to my hospital bed, I put my hands down at my sides and pushed my body up. What I didn't know was that there were five-foot-long clear plastic drainage tubes imbedded deeply in my face, neck, and shoulder, and that these were attached to an electric machine that suctioned lymphatic fluid and blood. And when I put my hands down and pressed my body up, I pulled all those strategically placed suction tubes out of the holes where my surgeon had carefully stitched them into place. Not a good thing. Especially since I had just had around two-hundred lymph nodes removed from my face, neck, and shoulder.

The lymph nodes' most significant purpose is to drain the lymphatic fluid that normally accumulates at a wound site after a serious injury or major surgery. The tubes had been put into place to suck out the rapidly accumulating lymphatic fluid, now that all the lymph nodes that controlled the swelling in that part of my body had been surgically removed. Since I no longer had lymph nodes in that part of my body or any properly seated plastic drainage tubes, in just a matter of hours my face and head swelled up to twice its normal size. I felt and looked like Mr. Potato Head.

Every couple of hours, a nurse or a doctor would come into my room and bury a big hypodermic needle deep into my face and neck to extract a large amount of fluid. This was done to help the swelling go down and reduce the chance of infection from all the stagnant fluid accumulating under the skin. The needle in the face would have bothered me except I was given a handheld remote that controlled a morphine device to help me with the pain. I had never before experienced a painkiller like morphine, and it is very powerful stuff. It's absolutely wonderful medicine in the right hands, and according to what I have read about it since then, patients who use it only for the reduction of postoperative pain rarely, if ever, get addicted to it.

My operation took more than eleven hours from start to finish. My surgeon was on his feet the entire time as he peeled back the left side of my face—like in the movie *Face/Off*—and carefully removed my left salivary gland (also known as the parotid gland) and the associated lymph nodes. That operation is called a radical parotidectomy. ("Radical," in a medical sense, refers to a surgical procedure associated with a malignancy.) Then he removed the left trapezoid muscle in my shoulder and neck, along with my left jugular vein and all the lymph nodes associated with that part of my body. That is called a radical neck dissection.

My left jugular vein—we all have one running up and down each side of our necks—was removed because there was a large lymph node resting directly on top of it that my doctors felt was very likely to be cancerous. It was virtually impossible to remove that node without removing the jugular vein as well, so it just had to go.

Finally, the surgeon removed a very large piece of my left ear, down to the earlobe. Removing such a large piece of my ear was essential because this was the site of the initial tumor, and the margins—the spaces between where the tumor was and where healthy normal tissue is—have to be significant, especially for a tumor as highly malignant as mine was. While I was still deeply anesthetized, the surgeon inserted numerous tubes to drain off the lymphatic fluid (to reduce swelling and the chance of infection), then tightly wrapped my head with sterile gauze, and covered that with a drab brown pressure dressing. He was done by dinnertime. He'd started around seven in the morning.

I remember almost nothing of day one. By day two I was no longer nauseated, but I could barely move because I was in so much pain. But then when I clicked on the morphine dispenser a few times, I drifted off into Never Never Land, until the pain rolled back an hour later. I could barely see because my face was so badly swollen. My eyes were slits.

But day three, when I had a moment all alone, I crawled out of bed and mustered up the courage to take a look at myself in the mirror. You see, it was Peggy's and my fourteenth wedding anniversary and I wanted to get prettied up for her arrival that morning. Wow—what a shock that was, peering into the mirror. From the end of my left shoulder to the top of my head, I was wrapped like a mummy in one continuous strand of two-inch-wide hospital gauze. Only my right eye and my nose were visible. The gauze was stained a deep brownish red from both dried and still wet blood. Clear plastic tubes and wires protruded from every part of my face and neck, most of them no longer properly drawing fluids, but sucking air instead, and making a horrendous noise to boot. My head had swelled up to a grand size. If Peggy could handle my looking like this on our fourteenth wedding anniversary, then she would be able to handle me if we were somehow blessed enough to grow old and gray and feeble together. At least that's what I was hoping.

When Peggy walked in, she gave me some colorful flowers, a long hug, and a tentative kiss, afraid she'd hurt the little bit of my face that was not stained with iodine or covered with elastic pressure dressing. She looked both spectacularly beautiful and as radiant as an angel to me. I swear it looked like she had a halo around her head, but maybe that had something to do with the morphine.

I told her how much I loved her and she told me the same, although Peggy has the uncanny ability to express a tremendous amount of love and emotion without saying very many words at all—one of her most endearing qualities. And I shared with her that no matter what happened, I wanted her to know that she was the greatest thing to ever happen to me and she was the most wonderful person to ever come into my life. We quietly reflected for a moment on how lucky we were to have found each other. Then Peggy and I set a simple and clear short-term goal for both of us to focus on: for me to be alive to celebrate our fifteenth wedding anniversary together.

A few hours later, we got a look at what was under the pressure dressing wrapped around my head, when my surgeon carefully removed the old bloodstained one and replaced it with a clean dressing. What a sight! Huge, long incisions all up and down and around my bright red swollen face, neck, and shoulder. It looked like hundreds of large, bright brass-colored staples were used to close those jagged incisions. But the puny remains of my left ear was the hardest thing for me to look at. "I hope we removed enough," the doctor said. "Me too," I responded, as I squirmed at my reflection in the mirror. "Finally I look like a movie star," I said to myself. "Boris Karloff."

The following day, I was released from the hospital. I won't ever forget how caring and supportive the doctors and nurses were during my stay with them. But I was very glad to be discharged because I'd found it almost impossible to get any sleep in the hospital. A hospital room has to be one of the noisiest and most disruptive places in the world. Don't ever go to a hospital to get some rest. Someone is always coming into your room just as you are about to fall asleep. It could be a nurse, a doctor, a janitor, a family member, or a friend. Even people you don't like can very easily stop in and visit you at the hospital, where you're a captive audience for their intrusive questions and stares. I couldn't wait to get home and into Peggy's and my own bed for a full night's sleep.

Using a wheelchair, Peggy and a nurse brought me down the hospital elevator to our car waiting out front. I was very heavily sedated but still conscious. Peggy and the nurse some-how helped me climb into the front passenger seat of our forest-green Plymouth Voyager. On the drive home, we stopped at a red light and I saw a car drive up and stop in the lane to the right of us. I must have been quite a sight, a bloody mummy peering, glassy-eyed, out the passenger side window at the older gentleman in the driver's seat of the car stopped next to us. Suddenly, the man stuck a lit cigarette in his mouth and took a long deep drag on it, closing his eyes as he did so, in sensual pleasure. Immediately, without even knowing why, I started to feel sick to my stomach. A moment later, the light turned green—and I did, too—as the old man with the ciga-rette in his mouth sped away.

Later, I wondered at my newly heightened sensitivity. I know that smoking does not have a direct causal effect on malignant melanoma. But somehow, the idea of anybody knowingly doing anything that causes cancer began to affect me in a very profound way.

I know that smoking does not cause malignant melanoma or a variety of other cancers. But I am quite certain that anyone who is dealing with malignant melanoma or another non-lung-type cancer who continues to smoke will dramatically compro-mise—even cripple—his or her immune system. And this will drastically raise the odds that the primary tumor will be able to migrate or metastasize to a distant part of the body and kill them. Loading up your blood with the carcinogens contained in cigarette smoke is probably one of the most powerful ways to destroy your immune system. And since cancer is caused primarily by a weakened immune system, the more you smoke, the more likely you will die from cancer, particularly as you and your immune system start to age.

So, something that was as meaningless to me in the past as

observing a stranger take a drag on a cigarette, suddenly, dramatically, had taken on a whole new meaning. I was reflecting on this, still doped up on morphine and exhausted from the lack of sleep during my hospital stay, as Peggy pulled into our driveway.

Once home, Peggy almost had to reintroduce me to the kids, I looked so different from the father they had said good-bye to just four days earlier. I remember green-eyed Christie had the cutest little brown leather cowgirl outfit on when she came into our bedroom holding hands with Peggy and Brian. Her eyes suddenly grew wide in amazement, especially after she heard a voice she recognized as mine coming from the mummylike figure before her. I was stained with iodine, and there was a tuft of blood-soaked hair popping out from under the pressure dressing at the top of my enormously swollen head. Brian asked to touch my head, then he said that I looked like a "Mummy-Daddy." We all laughed about that and it became Brian and Christie's new nickname for me around the house—Mummy-Daddy.

Word had gotten out among our friends that I was home recovering from the surgery, and I soon got a call from Dr. John Rossi and his wife, Roxanne. John was a veterinarian of significant renown in the area because he took excellent care not only of northern Florida's dogs and cats, he also handled exotic animals. His specialty was herpetology, the study of reptiles and amphibians, which are cold-blooded. People came from far and wide with their sick "herps" for him to care for. We'd met Dr. Rossi years earlier when we brought him a crippled six-foot-long red rat snake someone had shot with a pellet rifle. Sick pythons, pregnant tortoises, green iguanas with broken tails, giant toads with digestive problems—these are just a few of the bizarre problems Dr. Rossi has described in the several books he has authored on the unusual subject of herp husbandry. Dr. Rossi has more than earned the nickname the Cold-Blooded Vet, which his devoted patrons have bestowed upon him.

Dr. Rossi called soon after I got home from the hospital to tell me he had a favor to ask of me. It seemed that someone had brought to his office a tiny ball of fur that had fallen from a nest high above in an oak tree. And that ball of fur, about the size of a walnut, was alive. It was a baby flying squirrel, not yet weaned and just about to open its eyes. Dr. Rossi and his wife had nursed the little guy back to health. Now he needed a permanent home.

John felt that this tiny baby squirrel might be just the distraction—and just the medicine—that his sliced and diced morphine-addled friend might need to help him through his cancer challenge. Dr. Rossi didn't share any of those thoughts with me at the time, nor did he share with me how many times he has had to put down his clients' favorite pets because of skin cancer and melanomas, a not uncommon disease, particularly among older dogs and cats.

"John—yeah, sure, a pet flying squirrel—yeah, that would be really fun," I said to him on the phone.

"We'll bring it over later this afternoon," he replied. "Bill, wait till you see this little guy. He's really cute. He's just opened up his eyes."

A few minutes later, jokingly, I asked Peggy and the kids if they minded if another aviator came to live with us. Peggy gave me a questioning look; my bachelor Navy pilot buddies were the last people on earth she'd want living with us full-time. Some of them tended to be, well, just a tad wild.

When I told her the houseguest I was proposing was a tiny flying squirrel and not a Navy pilot, she and the kids were delighted. Always the animal lover, and especially a sucker for cute and cuddly baby animals, Peggy helped me set up a tall white birdcage in our kitchen for the furry little aviator's arrival.

Soon, this tiny furball was nestled in the chest pocket of my burgundy terry bathrobe, munching on a pecan, a favorite treat. As he stared up at me from the pocket of my robe with his enormously out-of-proportion jet-black eyes, it was easy to see how the southern flying squirrel ended up with the latin name *glaucomys*, which means "bulging eyes." This species' huge black eyes had evolved in a way that helps them see at night, the only time they are up and about. If they weren't nocturnal, they would be the meal of every hawk and snake in America. At night they normally have only owls to worry about, but for a wild flying squirrel, that's more than enough.

The smallest of the North American tree squirrels even when full grown, this baby squirrel, just a few months old, with its silky gray-brown-fur back and pure-white-furred belly was a joy to behold. I instantly connected with this tiniest of creatures. And it appeared that the feeling was mutual. He fell asleep in my bathrobe pocket as soon as he finished the pecan Christie had given him.

"What should we name him?" Peggy exclaimed. "Rocky!" Brian and Christie immediately cried out. Peggy, not a fan of such simple and obvious names for pets, tried to argue against it, but the twins' delight in what they thought was the best and most original name imaginable won out in just a few short minutes. I was in no shape to argue with them, and Rocky seemed an easy name to remember. I needed things to be easy right then.

After about an hour, Rocky woke and scampered to the top

of my head. He then peered down at my left ear as if to say, "Oh, boy, what happened to that?" He probably thought one of his larger cousins, a gray squirrel perhaps, had jumped out of a tree and chomped off my ear.

Rocky decided he liked it up on the top of my head, and almost every day he would sit up there, eat a pecan, and generally survey his squirreldom until he was ready for bed. At siesta time, Rocky sat on top of my scarred shoulder underneath my bathrobe or surrounded by fluffed-out cotton in the nest box in his cage, giving both of us a chance to catch up on some valuable time to reflect on our rather unique pasts.

I've always been an animal lover. Growing up, our house in northern New Jersey was perched midway up the side of a very steep and densely forested hill. Massive thick-stumped oak, hickory, and other deciduous trees of all types not only lined our street but grew haphazardly throughout the neighborhood, without any apparent organized thought by a city planner or the gentle touch of a gardener's green thumb. In that regard, God's thumb was certainly good enough, because living that close to nature was heaven to me.

The hundred-year-old homes appeared new to the area compared to the ancient trees that surrounded them. I loved those big old trees and the way they dominated the terrain, especially the huge, ancient oak in the yard next door. My brothers and sisters and I affectionately called it the Snake Tree.

Covered from top to bottom with thick, brown, musty-smelling vines that to us kids looked like a gigantic tower of snakes, it was the perfect tree for climbing up—way up—especially at night, to get a view of New York City's glorious skyline all lit up some thirty miles to the east.

Sometimes, while hanging on for dear life from the top of the Snake Tree, I swore I saw something small and ghostlike, like a pale gray Frisbee, flitting between the trees below, almost always in a straight line, always moving from a higher position to a lower position, shooting quickly down the steep incline in front of my family's three-story wood-shingled home. But when my eyes tried to follow this bizarre shadow-like thing from the point of takeoff to the point where it seemed to touch down—which was always another tree—there was nothing there to see. Nothing at all. Zero. It was just plain weird.

When I pointed out these curious sightings to my brothers and sisters and friends, they always told me the same thing: that I must have seen an owl, or a barn swallow, or a bat, or even a whippoorwill. But when I insisted I recognized full well what those creatures of the night looked like and it certainly wasn't one of them, I was told I must be seeing things—that my imagination must be getting the best of me.

And this was the thing they said that really got to me: that I should get my eyes checked—that I must be going blind.

Wrong. Wrong. Wrong. I knew my eyesight was exceptional, especially when I was out in the woods with my buddies Greg O'Neil, Chris McHugh, and Sandy North, also known as Rat, Cubie and Foof by the other kids in our neighborhood. Intensely curious about the wild world around us, we would methodically pick our way through the forest, climbing up trees to peer into bird and squirrel nests, curious to see if there were any new hatchlings or babies inside. And we would often foolishly stick our hands deep down inside dark holes under boulders and tree roots, hoping to grab hold of some yet undiscovered creature, furry or slimy (and hopefully not full of teeth), to examine and keep as a pet for a while. Then, after we had satisfied our curiosity, we made a concerted effort to release the animal exactly where we had found it. Why? Because I was a prodigious reader about wild animals, and that's what the books always said about wild things—to let them go exactly where you found them. And even as a small kid, I figured if someone picked me up in front of my home, I certainly wouldn't want them to drop me off, alone, in the center of New York City, and then assume I'd know how to take it from there.

Well, back to my eyesight. On our daily jaunts in the woods, Rat, Cubie and Foof were always commenting on how I spotted animals of all sorts well before they did, no matter how tiny or still or well camouflaged an animal appeared to be. Especially snakes.

Foof didn't like snakes. Rat and Cubie did. But I loved them. Unfortunately, my family did not share my enthusiasm. So I tested their patience, and I guess also their love, whenever they would discover some escaped serpent crawling out from under the television set while we watched it together after dinner. Or, much to their dismay, they would feel one of my critters slithering across the towel rack in the bathroom as they blindly reached for something to dry their eyes with after taking a shower. I wasn't the most popular member of the Goss household. You get the picture.

And even though I had this deep interest in snakes, I also had a deep interest and love for all of God's creatures, including rodents, and especially the type of gray squirrels common where we lived, so it pained me even to think about feeding my pet snakes the one rodent they required every month to survive. Thankfully I was able to persuade my smaller pet snakes to eat dead mice I bought frozen at the local pet store. I would also feed my six-foot-long black rat snake the occasional gray squirrel I would find dead on the road in front of our home. This earned me one of my many ignominious nicknames, Road Kill.

I had always been nuts for squirrels and I would catch them in a Havahart live-animal trap in our backyard just to get a chance to look at them up close for a few minutes. Then I'd let them go right where I caught them. Sometimes I was tempted to keep them longer, but my father, who was not a fan of gray squirrels (he favored the cute little red ones) would constantly remind me of how gray squirrels chewed hard-to-see holes high up under the eaves of old wooden homes like ours, allowing not only squirrels but birds and even bats to raise holy hell in the household.

So, as you can imagine, I had cages and aquariums full of all sorts of animals, semihidden in corners of my bedroom and in our basement. All things considered, I have to admit that my mother and father were quite tolerant of my many pets and everything that came with them. At the time, though, I didn't believe my parents had any tolerance at all. I usually had to beg and plead with Mom and Dad to add some new creature to my collection, often without success, so I usually just kind of sneaked the creatures into our house and then shot up the stairs, hiding each new pet as discreetly as possible under my shirt, regardless of how large or active an animal it was.

As my collection of critters grew, my eldest sister, Mimi, and my two older brothers, Bobby and Larry, all eventually moved into tiny rooms in the attic, claiming to want to get as far away as possible from the zoo in my bedroom. They had no desire, none at all, for one of my furred, feathered, or scaled friends to climb into bed and surprise them late at night while they were sound asleep, the sheets pulled up tight to their chins. But I believe it happened once or twice.

By the time I had reached double digits and Larry was thirteen, our family had pretty much adopted an old jet-black cat named Mischief, which another family in our neighborhood had kind of booted out. My father, who for some reason had a particular fondness for cats over dogs (he admired their independent streak), took pity and invited him in. One day I remember seeing Larry chasing Mischief through our backyard in a mad dash, something I had never seen Larry do before, and you have to believe I'd seen Larry do a lot of crazy things. So of course I took off in hot pursuit to see what was up. When I finally caught up with them, I discovered Larry on the ground, with Mischief on his lap, gently trying to persuade Mischief to release his grip on some small creature. Finally successful and without getting bitten, Larry said, "Here, Billy, take it quick—and get it away from Mischief!"

In my hands he placed an adorable little chipmunk that Larry would name—how original—Chipper.

Chipper was already almost full-grown. He was also hard to hold, lightning fast, and soon earned another nickname—Nipper.

My parents wisely encouraged us to give that little chipmunk another shot at freedom as soon as he was well enough to have a crack at that nut. We had simply gotten Chipper a little too late in his development for him to prefer domestic life over living wild and, being almost a teenager myself, I could relate to that. So we saved Chipper's life, nursed him back to health, and a few weeks later released him back to the wild, far away from his feline fan.

Of course, I missed Chipper and hated to see him go, but

he really was my brother Larry's pet, and by helping Larry care for him, I quickly learned many, but certainly not all, of the challenges associated with caring for a small but very alert and extremely fast-moving creature.

Because I was so attached to Chipper and was somewhat brokenhearted when we set him free, my parents surprised me that Christmas with another cute and cuddly rodent just about the size of a chipmunk. But this adorable little creature was a native of a country on the other side of the world.

Ginger was the world's cutest little golden hamster, a nocturnal burrowing animal native to the deserts of Syria. Someone a long time ago decided to bring a box of them to the United States and start breeding them for research and for pets. And breed they did. There are millions and millions of hamsters now in research facilities, pet stores, and in homes across America. Much slower-moving than the squirrels and chipmunks I was used to, Ginger used to spend half the day in my shirt pocket, asleep most of the time, because of his habitual late-night carousing on his exercise wheel. I remember my father reminding me time and time again to oil that exercise wheel so it wouldn't make that irritating noise in the middle of the night, kind of like the sound of chalk on a very dry blackboard (soon to be followed by an even worse noise: "Billy! Will you shut that hamster the hell up!").

Of course, I never used oil on Ginger's wheel for fear he would lick it off and get sick, or even die. I used butter or margarine instead, which didn't work nearly as well as lubricating oil, because Ginger would lick it off the axle faster than you can say Blue Bonnet. Which, of course, would get that darn exercise wheel squealing again like a stuck pig.

Ginger thrived on a diet that many small rodents seem to

enjoy: sunflower seeds and nuts of all kinds, carrots, apples, and other fresh fruits and vegetables. He also liked a salted cracker with peanut butter, as well as a dried chicken bone to gnaw on. The chicken bone was a good source of calcium for Ginger. It was especially helpful in sharpening his front teeth and wearing them down. Otherwise, his incisors might have grown so long that he wouldn't be able to use them anymore.

Now, there are a couple of things you should know about Ginger. First, Ginger was a secondhand hamster. I didn't mind. When you're the fourth of six children, pass-me-downs are the rule, not the exception. It seemed somebody's little princess had lost interest in the cuddly baby girl hamster that she had named Ginger. The little girl and her parents now wanted Ginger out of their lives forever. So my parents, knowing that *their* son would never lose interest in a pet and was looking for a new furry little animal to call his own, easily persuaded the girl's parents not to drown Ginger in a bucket of water, as had been suggested, but instead to give her another chance at life in *our* house—as long, of course, as the cage, food, water bottle, exercise wheel, etc., were thrown in for good measure, preferably just before Christmas. My parents weren't stupid—they knew how to strike a good deal. Even over a rodent. But with six kids closely spaced in age all living under one roof, Barbara and Gene just didn't want to be burdened with too many details.

So it was I who discovered, relatively quickly I might add for a young boy, that the rapidly maturing Ginger was a not a *she*—but instead was a *he*—"not that there's anything wrong with it." And as young hamsters grow and sexually mature, they grow a set of gonads so large it would be obvious to even the most uninitiated that *she* was a *he*. It's probably something the little girl's parents discovered just a few days before striking the Christmas rodent deal with my parents. Timing *is* everything. My family tried to get me to change his name to something a little more manly, like Manster. It had a nice ring to it. Manster the Hamster. But I wouldn't have it. I just didn't want to mess up my little hamster's head any more than was absolutely necessary. Ginger would have more than enough to deal with, just living with the rest of the Goss clan.

What an unbelievable Christmas that was for me. My parents successfully hid Ginger until I thought the last gift had been handed out. Then Mom and Dad uncovered Ginger's cage and told me she—I mean he—was mine. Secondhand or not, Ginger was the greatest. We had wonderful fun together, although he occasionally escaped from his cage, especially at night, when these nocturnal critters are most active.

I remember one occasion when, deep in the middle of the night, I heard my father yell out my name in his deep, powerful voice.

"Billlly!"

I thought I was dreaming. "Billlly . . ." There, like a foghorn, I thought I heard it again. This time I did wake up and shot out of bed. "This can't be good for anyone," I said to myself, " . . . especially me."

Evidently my parents had been awakened by a very mysterious rustling sound coming from the corner of their bedroom. When my father, half-asleep, finally pinpointed the location of the noise, he was surprised to discover it coming from his briefcase.

Evidently Ginger had climbed in a few hours earlier and had decided to take an important business report my father had written earlier that evening and start shredding it with his teeth to prepare a nest. Maybe marking my territory wouldn't be such a bad idea either, Ginger must have thought to himself, as he sprayed his scent over my dad's documents, to warn any other carousing hamsters from entering Ginger's newfangled den. With the shredding job nearly complete, Ginger had a nice soft place to curl up and sleep after a hard night's work. The sun would be rising in just an hour or two. Ginger was tired. I mean, really, a hamster needs its rest too. But then Ginger heard the sound of a potentially deadly predator: "Billlly!"

Well, as you can imagine, it took a lot of explaining, pleading, begging, and cajoling to persuade my father to let me keep Ginger. And keep him I did—Ginger lived to be almost five years old, a very ripe age for a pet hamster, or any other small animal for that matter.

Maybe this was just a start—a start in discovering the secret to longevity. I hoped I'd now get to apply some of this rodent longevity knowledge with Rocky, as he grew from a boy into a man.

Over the course of the next few weeks, on a diet of nuts, fruits, mixed bird seed, and vegetables, Rocky grew from the size of a single walnut to the size of a bar of soap, about four or even six walnuts in size, collectively.

One morning, while I was reading the *Florida Times-Union* with Rocky perched on top of my head, busily grooming himself, I raised a cup of coffee to my lips with my right hand while I continued to hold the newspaper with my left. Peggy and the twins were running around the kitchen getting ready for school. Suddenly: "Ah-chooooo!" I closed my eyes and sneezed with all my might. Nicely recovering from the sneeze, still holding my coffee with my right hand in front of my face, I again tilted the cup up against my lips. To my amazement, staring directly at me were Rocky's two huge eyes, now with his front little feet perched on the edge of the cup, as if he were kneeling in prayer, perhaps praying to get out of this unlikely predicament.

"There's a squirrel in my coffee!" I cried out in utter amazement to Peggy and the kids.

Like a flash, Rocky shot out of the cup and onto my shoulder, and then, with one more leap, up to the top of my head again. I could feel him preening himself, licking the coffee from his drenched fur like there was no tomorrow. What a caffeine buzz Rocky was going to get, I thought.

But then I had another thought, and it was this: Lately I had been feeling a bit sorry for myself. Maybe I was feeling a little bit of "Why me, God? Why did you give me cancer at only thirty-eight years of age? What did I do wrong? Wasn't I among your chosen—don't I count—aren't I one of your more unique creations?"

The answer was forthcoming, a truly profound realization for me, inspired by Rocky's dip in my coffee. God wanted me to know that of course I was unique. Because I absolutely, positively had to be the only person in the world—out of the 6 billion or more people walking the face of the earth at any given moment—who had a flying squirrel in his coffee that morning. Damn right that made me unique. Damn right that made me special.

And sometimes it is that feeling of being unique, of being special and one with God, particularly when you're reflecting on the immensity and infinite nature of the universe, that takes away the sense of aloneness, and of being separate and unconnected to the universe. Feeling unique can make all the difference in a person's outlook about getting well again. It can help to supercharge your human spirit, help to kick it into afterburner.

Especially for a guy like me, a Navy pilot, with a tiny little furball of an angel not yet qualified to fly, serving as my new copilot.

6

What Makes Rocky Unique

*R*ocky quickly became an important part of the Goss family. Besides continuing to learn more about cancer, I now wanted to learn as much as possible about flying squirrels in general, and about Rocky in particular. You see, I no longer wanted to lick my own wounds, so to speak. I wanted to make sure I was taking the best possible care of this tiny, hapless little aviator who fell out of the sky and into my life just when I needed him most. He deserved the best. I was going to get him into top shape—even though he weighed in at only one ounce when he first took up residence in the corner of our kitchen.

Rocky also proved to be the perfect distraction as I weaned myself off the postsurgery morphine and codeine and the other painkillers I had been prescribed. I just wanted to start getting high on life itself, especially since I'd gotten such a clear and frightening look at the alternative. High on life itself . . . it sounds so cliché, so seventies, so unlike anything I would ever say now. But no other words can explain the transformation I underwent with my fellow aviator Rocky as a copilot—and my family and friends as members of my flight crew—as I began to look at the world from a whole new point of view, like from high up in an airplane, where everything just looks so beautiful.

After doing extensive research on the Internet and at the library, on both cancer and flying squirrels, I thought I had learned enough to give Rocky a pretty good shot at living a long and happy life. A long and happy life measured in squirrel years, of course. Unfortunately, in talking with zoologists and veterinarians, I found that a squirrel year, unlike a dog or cat year (one human year equals seven dog or cat years), has yet to be accurately determined. And when I'd asked them to be a little bit more specific, if they could provide me with a formula for figuring out not only flying squirrel years, but more specifically southern flying squirrel years, I'd get a rather curious look from them. But one thing they all agreed on was this: The "average" life span of a wild flying squirrel, from birth to death, is a very short period of time. One, maybe two years at max. Because, from the moment a baby flying squirrel is born, usually in the late spring, the odds are stacked way against it.

After a forty-day gestational period, baby flying squirrels come into the world tiny, naked, hairless, and blind, usually with four or five siblings. Typically they are born in a hole hollowed out by a woodpecker high up in a dead tree or in a small nest made out of leaves and twigs and moss. Baby flying squirrels have zero defenses in the first few months of life except the innate protectiveness of their mother, who weighs just a few ounces herself. For a baby flying squirrel, surviving long enough to get in that first flight, their solo, is more than just luck, it's almost a miracle.

Getting wet from the rain and dying from hypothermia, getting blown to the ground on a windy day, besides crows, blue jays, and many other hungry birds snapping them up as a snack, survival for a baby flying squirrel is almost a living hell. There are also tree-climbing snakes, raccoons, gray squirrels, bobcats, house cats, and virtually any other animal that wants a little additional protein in its diet, to add to this list of predators. With their biggest threat of all being owls—especially the huge and immensely powerful great horned owl—baby flying squirrels have almost no chance of making it to sexual maturity and an even slimmer chance of living a full adult life.

And don't forget—somewhere in there, during their flying squirrel teenage years, they have to squeeze in attending flight school, and that carries a very high rate of mortality in and of itself. Just like when I was in pilot training in Texas. I lost several friends, all of them in their early twenties, killed in Navy flight training accidents. Many years earlier, during WWI, my grandfather Pop Dacey also attended pilot training in Texas. Soon after he soloed, Pop accompanied his best friend back to see his parents in their home state of Massachusetts. Unfortunately, Pop's friend made the trip beside him in a pine casket. Learning to conquer the air, for humans, and probably even more so for flying squirrels, can sometimes be a very dangerous proposition.

My first solo took place in a Navy North American T-28 Trojan. After twelve flights with an instructor, I was at last ready to solo in the gigantic 1,425-horsepower radial-engine airplane. Here I was in an airplane ten times more powerful than the plane in which most people typically solo. It was deafeningly loud, and *very* intimidating to fly. Frankly, I was scared to death of flying it alone and for the first time. On takeoff, if you add power to the massive engine too quickly without applying a lot of rudder pedal with your right foot, the T-28 would do a torque roll right there on the runway, flipping upside down on top of you, crushing the glass canopy—and the pilot—underneath its 8,500 pounds. It was a big, scary beast, that airplane, but I wanted to do it so badly I could almost taste it. Many student pilots shared that feeling. We weren't afraid of flying, we were just afraid of flying the T-28 Trojan. It's weird and unnatural to be motivated toward something you fear, but that's just the way it is in flight school.

But let's get back again to flying squirrels in general. First, there are only two species of flying squirrels in North America. The slightly larger and darker brown northern flying squirrel, Latin name *Glaucomys sabrinus*, weighs in at a whopping four to six ounces and stretches a massive ten to twelve inches from the tip of its nose to the end of its bushy, flat, rudderlike tail. Northern flying squirrels are found throughout Canada, New England, and the Pacific Northwest.

Rocky is a southern flying squirrel, *Glaucomys volans*, the slightly smaller, grayer, and (as some zoologists and keepers of exotic pets have stated) *friendlier* squirrel, found generally to the south of his northern cousin. Southern flying squirrels weigh in at two to three ounces and stretch out from nose to tail at about nine to ten inches. They are generally found in the states bordering or east of the Mississippi River.

Obviously, I was surprised to learn that the ghostlike creatures that made me think I was seeing things as a boy growing up in New Jersey were not northern flying squirrels, but instead were the southern variety. I learned that the word *southern*, when it's used in conjunction with the two species of flying squirrels in North America, means south of the Canadian border, not south of the Mason-Dixon Line.

Rocky turned out to be a spectacularly fun-loving and adorable pet who felt particularly comfortable around me—my voice, my heartbeat, even my smell—as he ate pecans on top of my head during my morning newspaper and coffee. Getting Rocky right after he opened his eyes allowed a powerful bond to develop between us. Actually, according to animal behaviorists, I technically imprinted myself on Rocky as his parent. He opened his eyes, heard my voice, saw my face, and thought, "Mama." In some ways, Rocky is probably more comfortable with me, a human being, than he would be with another flying squirrel. We've developed a wonderful relationship, unlike any I've had with other animals. And I've had a lot of special relationships with many other of God's creatures.

Rocky is the same species as the supercool and ultrahip flying squirrel made famous by the original Rocky and Bullwinkle cartoons, with their perpetual evil antagonists, Boris, Natasha, and Fearless Leader. Flying squirrels in the wild prefer living in and around deciduous or mixed deciduous-coniferous trees. They are North America's only strictly nocturnal squirrels. In Rocky's case, this never changed. He started out and stayed a real night owl, no matter how hard we tried to get him to go diurnal for us. Living in our kitchen, Rocky waits up to see us in the early morning as the twins, Brian and Christie, get ready for school and Peggy and I get ready for the day's events.

You cannot believe how my heart melted when tiny Rocky was placed in my hands. How taken I was when Rocky would peek up into my eyes from deep inside my shirt pocket. Especially when he'd start chirping at me in a scolding fashion, demanding I get him another pecan from our kitchen pantry.

During breakfast we lean from the kitchen table to give him a raisin from our granola or a piece of banana, melon, or even a blueberry or a strawberry as a special treat. Flying squirrels enjoy all forms of nuts, fruits, mushrooms, lichen, seeds, and even an occasional crunchy insect.

In captivity as well as in the wild, dietary calcium and salt are vital for their survival. When you find shed deer antlers or an animal skeleton while hiking in the woods, you'll often see that they have been nibbled on by wild flying squirrels in their constant efforts to get calcium and salt. They also glide onto backyard bird feeders, sometimes accounting for significant losses of bird food throughout the night.

Rocky often stays awake long enough to watch all four of us have breakfast together—all five of us if you include Rocky's buddy, Peanut, our wonderful little Yorkshire terrier, or Yorkie as they are commonly called.

Each morning and evening, Peanut, all five pounds of her, trots over to Rocky's little white house to say hello. They kiss nose to nose. Then, if Rocky is in a good mood, he will chirp excitedly—birdlike, like a warbler—and sprint up and down and all around his cage, getting Peanut more and more excited. This continues until Peanut starts barking in response to Rocky's high-pitched twittering, and soon a real cross-species conversation—I guess you could even call it an argument—ensues.

Sometimes, if they really start getting crazy with each other, I'm forced to yell, "Hey! Cut it out!" especially if one of us is in the kitchen trying to talk on the phone. This command usually causes them both to stop immediately, but then they repeat the same wildly hysterical scene the following evening.

This kind of hyperkinetic activity occurs every night, all year long. Unlike a lot of other animals, woodchucks for instance, flying squirrels do not hibernate, and remain fully energized even during the coldest weather. When a bad winter snowstorm strikes, several, sometimes as many as twenty, will move in together in a hollow tree to share body heat and swap flying stories.

Even in the dead of a winter's night, they actively glide from tree to tree, using the skin between their forelegs and hind legs. This skin, a combination parachute and sail, along with their rudderlike tails for steering, allows flying squirrels to turn and change their angle of descent quite dramatically throughout their glides.

As agile, sure-footed, and confident as flying squirrels are while sprinting up tree trunks and when jumping out airborne in a glide like some kind of wacky extreme sport—like base jumping—they appear quite awkward when trying to run across a horizontal surface. But they're still tough to catch when on the ground because their movements are so erratic and they're so darn small. Generally, it seems to me, flying squirrels prefer to travel by air rather than ground transportation, much like modern-day human travelers.

When Rocky leaps from my shoulder to Peggy's shoulder and then to Brian's head, he seems like he's king of the world. But if he jumps from Brian to Christie and misjudges the distance, only to land on our hardwood floor with a resounding *splat*, Rocky looks stunned, like both his pride and his feelings have been hurt. After a questioning pause, he'll sprint to the nearest vertically rising object, usually one of our legs, shoot again to the top of someone's head, and start the whole game all over again. Leaping from one head to another is one of Rocky's favorite things to do, especially at night, when he's most active and alert. The evening hours are definitely when Rocky comes to life.

Late one night, I was awakened by an excessive amount of chirping and twittering going on in the kitchen. Peggy gave me a hug, then a poke, and while still asleep she softly said, "Could you get Rocky to quiet down, please?" Even Peanut, from her bed in the corner of our room, gave me a look like, "Heh, Dad, enough's enough." I climbed out of bed and went to look at Rocky. He was in his little white house on the top shelf of his tall cage, which sits next to a large window overlooking our backyard.

Rocky, perched in the corner of his cage, was looking out the window and chirping away like crazy. To my amazement, the reason his birdlike twittering sounded twice as loud as normal was because on the other side of the window, pressed up against the glass, was another flying squirrel, a wild one that evidently had climbed down from the large oak tree that emerges from the center of the wood deck behind our house. Ignoring my presence, Rocky and the wild flying squirrel continued their squirrel talk. I just didn't have the heart to break it up. That wild flying squirrel came down from the oak tree several more times to bring Rocky up-to-date on the latest in flying squirrel current events, probably discussing things like this year's acorn harvest, when animals attack, crash-landings into the sides of garages, and more.

Then one night Rocky's wild friend visited no more. Maybe a hungry owl had got him. I felt a pang of heartbreak for Rocky and had wanted to let him go run with the wolves, so to speak, but I knew he didn't stand a chance of surviving in the wild. He couldn't glide worth a damn and had not a clue that as soon as he landed on a tree he had to sprint around to the opposite side to avoid getting picked off by an owl.

For all I know, Rocky may have been telling the outside squirrel, "Hey, come in here. It's warm, and fun, and I get all the fresh food and water I want. I even get to eat pecans on top of this big animal's head every morning . . . he's a real dork."

Rocky's a character. Besides the special bond we share and his dynamic and constantly changing personality, what makes him so unique in the animal world is the folded layer of loose skin along each side of his body, from front leg to hind leg. This is found in no other mammal in North America except bats. Flying squirrels jump from tall trees and spread out all four legs as widely as possible to glide down to the trunks of other trees in the distance, sometimes as far as 250 feet away. They are North America's only true gliding mammal. Bats, another unique, kindred spirit of the night sky, are the only mammals in the world that can truly fly, maintaining level flight for an extended period of time like birds and insects do.

So what's the big difference between gliding and flying? When a flying squirrel jumps from a tree, spreads the loose folds of skin under its legs and starts gliding to another tree, he's always going down, like a single-engine airplane that's had a complete engine failure. A flying squirrel has an aerodynamic glide ratio dependent on several things. These include: the lift-generating capacity of the airfoil (the spread skin and body), along with its angle of attack, its speed through the air, and its weight, among other factors.

It's because a flying squirrel is so light and can spread its feet out into something that looks like a gray fur-lined Frisbee with a flat tail as a rudder for steering, combined with its courage to jump boldly into the night, that makes it, well, a flying squirrel. But, technically speaking, it shouldn't be called a flying squirrel. It should be called a gliding squirrel.

Let's freeze-frame at the end of a long glide. One second before a flying squirrel crashes itself headfirst into the side of a tree trunk at about thirty mph, it bends its flat rudderlike tail from a position horizontal to the ground to a position vertical to the ground. This causes the rest of the squirrel's body to suddenly flare upward and also causes the squirrel's gliding speed to dramatically slow down, its tail working like the speed brake on the bottom of the T-28 Trojan aircraft I used to fly.

And, in another way, it's almost identical to what I did as a Navy pilot when landing on a long runway. Just seconds before the wheels of the P-3 Orion I was flying were about to touch down, I would gently ease back on the four power throttles and even more gently pull back on the aircraft's yoke. This "flare" would rapidly slow the airplane's rate of descent and also its forward speed.

If I did it perfectly, which I've got to tell you wasn't too often, it would provide a smooth landing and a relatively slow touchdown speed, just like a perfect touchdown for a flying squirrel. The only difference being this: After I made a perfect landing I would wait to hear applause from my copilot and crew members—a flying squirrel is afforded no such luxury. The instant a flying squirrel touches down, it must immediately dash around to the opposite side of the tree. Any flying squirrel that does not do this does not live long. They do this so that any owl that may be in hot aerial pursuit during the squirrel's glide—a glide that may take several seconds and cover a couple of hundred feet in distance—is sorely disappointed when it gets to the landing zone and not a squirrel is there to be found.

This is also why it was so hard for my siblings and me to

realize that there were flying squirrels zipping back and forth from the giant oaks in our front yard to the towering elms in the neighboring yard. I'd see a ghostlike Frisbee shooting through the dark. I'd exclaim to my brothers and sisters, "Look—what's that?" And then I'd point to the tree where this thing flew to . . . and nothing would be there to show for it. What I didn't know then is that all I had to do was to look up the other side of the tree, and there it would be—a dark little form scampering straight to the top, a night paratrooper ready for another exhilarating jump into the darkness.

Darkness for us, I might say. With the jet-black, goggle-like eyes flying squirrels have, which are perfect for seeing at night (like the specially designed night-vision goggles I sometimes wore while flying Navy aircraft), an adult flying squirrel's night vision—along with its depth perception, coordination, and balance—must be extraordinary to avoid deadly high-speed crashes into the sides of trees. Yet, through the years, although I've happened upon countless dead gray squirrels, I have never—not even once—come upon a dead flying squirrel, adding to the intrigue of this somewhat mysterious little creature.

So be ready. Some night real soon, you might think your eyes are playing tricks on you when you see something that looks like the shadow of a Frisbee glide toward a tree near you and then suddenly disappear. If you're fast enough and smart enough to immediately shine a flashlight up the tree trunk opposite the side on which it landed, you might, just for a brief moment, see two bouncing reddish orange spots, before, in a snap, they disappear.

It's the reflection—the eyeshine—from the eyes of a wild flying squirrel that just happened to look down at you for a second, before heading up to the top of the tree again.

Consider yourself lucky. You've just seen something that happens many times each night, but is rarely observed by human eyes.

You've witnessed a visit from one of God's little angels, falling to earth like a tiny shooting star, before returning to the heavens again.

7

The Rocky Road to Recovery

*A*fter Rocky fell into my coffee, I continued to feel more and more inspired to get better—and even look better—as fast as humanly possible. Rocky was my copilot, my wingman, if you will. Nesting in my hair, perched like a king on his throne, staring down at my missing left ear like a missing left wing after an unlucky aerial dogfight, he must have wondered a bit at how he would get this thing, me, back together again in time for a safe landing. Unfortunately, that left wing—I mean ear, was not to be replaced soon. I was told by the hospital that I would have to remain cancer-free for at least one year before they would consider reconstructive surgery.

They weren't being cruel; they were being practical. If I had a recurrence, I would most likely need to have radiation treatment on my face, neck, and shoulder to slow the spread of the cancer. And any recent plastic surgery would be damaged by the radiation. In fact, a lot of the living tissue used in the reconstruction would die, leaving me even more scarred than before. And if I did have a recurrence, my chances of long-term survival would be very reduced, possibly making the plastic surgery a moot point, a waste of time for both my doctors and myself.

The Navy was kind enough, though, to pay for a pink rubber (well, actually silicone) prosthetic ear that I attached to the left side of my head with a Duco Cement–like substance. This lasted a very short period of time, however, because the silicone ear looked like the foreign thing that it was, like a tiny albino bat hitching a ride on the side of my head. Peggy, Brian, Christie, and Rocky found the whole thing rather frightening to look at. So, I grew my hair long around the ears, rather unmilitary-looking for a Navy pilot, but understandable by those who knew what I was going through.

When Rocky played on my head and neck and even slept on my scars under my bathrobe, at first, when I closed my eyes, I only knew when he was on the right side of my head and neck. I had no feeling on the left side at all. Also, I couldn't smile at first, because so many nerves on the left side of my face had been severed during the radical parotidectomy. But, because I was able to move my lips into an O shape, I was told that if I was lucky, enough nerves in my face had survived, and with some steady electrical-stimulation treatment, the cut nerves would be able to regenerate enough to let me at least crack a smile. Not a big smile, but a smile nonetheless.

The hospital loaned me a pocket stimulation device to shock my face in an attempt to slowly get my smile back.

Rocky once jumped onto my head from our kitchen table—my face already wired up and fired up and set to shock me every five seconds. Let me tell you, Rocky didn't like that thing one bit. I guess it also electrified my hair and my scalp, because Rocky almost took another nosedive into my coffee cup. But as the days progressed, so did my smile, with the help of my daily electroshock facial. And Rocky learned to avoid the top of my head when my face was wired up.

A few weeks after my surgery, more good news. The Armed Forces Institute of Pathology had examined all the lymph nodes that had been removed. Their findings were excellent. No gross tumors (I believe doctors use the word *gross* to mean visibly obvious tumors) in any of the lymph nodes, even the large inflamed node that had been wrapped around my left jugular vein, forcing my surgeon to remove that very significant source of blood flow to my brain.

The AFIP did not rule out the likelihood that there were microscopic cancer cells in the nodes they examined. But no obvious tumors in my lymph nodes—well, that was just great news.

My hilarious buddy Greg "Rat" O'Neil had flown in from Ohio with the single-minded goal of making me laugh for three days straight. He was successful. As he flew out of town, my brother Larry flew in to take over. When I asked Larry how I should celebrate the news that the lymph nodes they had removed were negative for cancer, he responded simply, "Buy a Porsche."

"What are you talking about, Larry?" I asked.

"Have you ever owned a nice sports car, Bill?"

"No."

"Well, don't you think now is as good a time as any? Don't you think you've earned it? Don't you think you deserve one?"

"Since you put it that way, yes, maybe I do."

"Well, then, let's go shopping."

I ended up buying a used Porsche in mint condition at a rock-bottom price. A gorgeous and very rich-looking silvery gray machine, I call it the Gray Ghost, which is also the nickname of my favorite bird of prey, the goshawk.

And the license plate I got with it? It reads: GOSHAWK.

Larry was right—I feel good every time I climb into that finely tuned automobile. If a cancer survivor wants to treat him- or herself to a fine ride, even as fine a ride as a Porsche, then they should go out there and get one. I've got to tell you this one more time because I'm dead serious: Every time I climb into that car, I feel good.

Because most of my left ear and left jugular vein were gone, I obviously had reduced value to the Navy as a pilot. The paperwork went into the system for me to receive a medical retirement. An enlisted person who later attains a commission as an officer in the United States Navy is referred to as a "mustang" (I have no idea where that expression came from), and that is what I was—a mustang. Because of the additional six years I had served as a Navy mine man prior to receiving my officer's commission, I was only months away from the twenty-year mark for military retirement.

I had always wanted to retire before my fortieth birthday. I just never thought—never imagined—it would be with a medical retirement due to cancer. Life is constantly throwing curve balls at us. I guess that's what makes life so interesting and exciting, so colorful and dramatic. And even fun, after you get through all the hard stuff.

After weaning myself off the morphine, then codeine, and then the super-duper 800 mg capsules of Tylenol, I started going out in public more often, which at first I had avoided because I didn't particularly enjoy grossing people out with my swollen and cut-up face, a big chunk of my left ear missing, and a bunch of scabs and scars from hell.

Yet, something interesting took place. It seemed my scars began to heal at an accelerated rate after I stopped taking medication for the pain. And, with the help of my family and friends, especially those with aviation inclinations like Rocky, I started getting physically stronger in many ways rather unusual for a man about to turn forty.

At about this time, I started working on my first book, *The Luckiest Unlucky Man Alive*. When did I initially get the writing bug? Well, ten years earlier, while a Navy pilot on my first tour of duty, I won the Navy Pilot Writer of the Year Award for a rather comprehensive aviation article I wrote for the prestigious naval aviation magazine *Approach*. The article I wrote was titled "Pilot in Command vs. Pilot at the Controls." It was about a major crash landing at an airport in Spain of a new $65 million Navy spy plane that I was in command of at the time, although I was not the pilot "at the controls" physically flying the aircraft. At least I thought I was in command of that airplane.

Luckily, no one was hurt, but the crash was a rather traumatic experience for a proud young Navy pilot who still had a lot to learn about personal humility and professional accountability. So this valuable lesson was delivered to me in one fell swoop. Writing the article helped me to put the whole experience into proper perspective, which in a nutshell was this: that my crew and I were lucky—really lucky—that nobody was killed or even hurt, which is the normal occurrence in a major crash landing. Writing the article helped other military pilots learn some valuable lessons about flying large and complex craft under simulated emergency conditions. That's probably why my piece won an award.

But most of all, writing that article helped put that tough challenge behind me so I could move forward with the rest of my life and career.

So I might have already had a little skill at writing. But my motivation for writing *The Luckiest Unlucky Man Alive* was entirely different. I started writing it at first to have something to leave my young children as a memoir so they would know who their dad was, just in case things didn't have the happy ending I was hoping for.

But, like writing about the plane crash, something positive started to happen to me as I recollected the many crazy friends I had and the many crazy things we'd done together. I truly believe that writing first helps the author by serving as a stress reliever for an overly wound-up brain, then it helps the reader. And I think, in my case anyway, that reviewing and reflecting on my life's many misadventures actually made me laugh as I relived this stuff in my mind while putting it down on paper, often serving as a huge boost to the cancer-fighting aspects of my immune system.

Reflecting on and writing about my past reduces stress and makes me laugh and smile. It's just what the doctor ordered. Just like Rocky.

A few months after my surgery, the deep scars on my neck no longer looked raw and red. But they were still ugly. More important, these scars had tightened up the left side of my neck so much that I couldn't turn my head to the left or right without very significant discomfort. And this wasn't a good thing, because one of your primary duties as a Navy pilot is to keep your head and eyes moving from side to side, like on a swivel, visually scanning your airspace to avoid a midair collision with another fast-moving craft, or with a tall building, radio tower, or mountain.

I talked about this with the head of ENT at the Navy hospital, a wonderful surgeon named Dr. Jeff Sandler. He looked at me and proposed he do a Z-plasty and dermabrasion on my major scars to loosen up my skin so that I would have improved flexibility in my head and neck. It might even improve my appearance, too. So a few days later I was under his scalpel. First, Dr. Sandler cut something like a Z, like the sign of Zorro, into the long, vertical ear-to-shoulder scar on my left side. The large Z cut was to provide a springlike incision to help unbind the tightness in my radical neck-dissection scar. After that, he applied something that looked and felt like a Craftsman belt sander to my neck to abrade (really more like sand down) the thick keloid scars that had developed, now, into something bloody and icky, but that would be much smoother and more flexible skin after it healed.

When I got home and Rocky took one look at this bloody mess, he decided to sleep on the top of my head, and not on top of these fresh scars under my bathrobe. He waited a few weeks until the skin had healed.

One thing that happens after you have a salivary gland removed is that for quite a period of time afterward, you drool. But you don't drool through your mouth, as you normally would, but instead you drool through the deep surgical incisions behind your ear and under your chin. This is apparently because the remaining part of your salivary system starts working overtime making saliva, and because saliva has so many powerful digestive enzymes in it, it prevents the surgical incisions from healing.

And when I smelled food, wow! The remaining salivary system would kick into overdrive, and drool would start flowing down my chin like a torrent, then drip onto my lap— causing me to be the brunt of many crude jokes from my family and friends. But every joke put a crooked smile on my face—each day my smile was getting a little straighter, so "a little less crooked" might be a better way of describing it—and my drooling was becoming a little less obvious. Faster and faster, I was healing.

Before I even knew I had cancer, I had agreed to go whitewater rafting down the Colorado River through some major rapids in the upper Grand Canyon over the course of a five-day trip. Jeff Marcketta and Dave Graziano, two of my very best buddies from grade school, were dumbfounded when I announced I'd still be making the trip with them. My head was still badly swollen and scraggly scars crawled down my neck, much like the river itself appeared as it carved its way along the Utah desert floor beneath the little airplane in which we were flying.

With the ice-cold river, the steaming sun, and the ice-cold beer, this seemed to me the perfect way to stave off postoperative depression—something I had been warned about by my doctors and nurses. The intense desert sun was probably not the best thing in the world for a melanoma patient, but with a long-sleeved shirt and pants, a big broad-rimmed hat, and plenty of sunscreen, I must have looked like one of the yahoos right out of the movie *Deliverance*. But I followed the cardinal rules about skin cancer prevention anyway: Slip, Slap, Slop: slip on a shirt, slap on a hat, and slop on some sunscreen.

Gliding down that roaring river, watching golden eagles and peregrine falcons soar along the Utah mountain ridges, was absolutely breathtaking. And for long spells on the river, I was lost in the grandeur of it all, this spectacular gift of earth and heaven combined, with two of my closest friends. For long periods of time I didn't feel any pain at all, just a oneness with the canyon and sheer exhilaration that comes from shooting down some of the biggest whitewater rapids in North America.

When I got home, I started looking in the real estate section of the *Florida Times-Union*, the largest newspaper in northeast Florida. I wanted to find a really rural kind of place, in a seriously wild setting like I had just enjoyed in Utah, to allow me to spend more time in the woods with Mother Nature. Peggy, wonderful Peggy, said fine. We'd look for it together.

It didn't take long before we found what we were looking for—a remote cabin on a large wilderness lake in Osceola National Forest connected to the world-famous Okefenokee Swamp. One of the reasons the Okefenokee is so well known is because it's the make-believe home of the comic strip character Pogo, the socially minded possum. This part of Florida and Georgia was loaded with wildlife, especially possums, though I don't remember any of them talking to me . . . at least I don't think I remember that.

However, when I was a kid I had two small baby possums my father found in the backyard for me early one morning before he left for work. For a few weeks, they sat on my head as I rode my bicycle around the neighborhood, much to the chagrin of the local moms, because they looked almost exactly like large rats. I think my dad got in trouble for that one. Anyway, one day Dad told me they were no longer in their cage in the backyard and must have gotten away. My mother's fear of my or my siblings contracting rabies from all these critters—a legitimate fear, I might add—probably led my father to release Abbott and Costello back into the wild.

Possums are not the smartest or friendliest of animals—in fact they have a perpetually ticked-off look on their faces—but they're North America's only true marsupial and only mammal with a prehensile tail. So, particularly as a young boy, they were very interesting to me in their own special way. This was also just another example of my father and mother encouraging me to be interested in what I was interested in—and not necessarily in what they were interested in.

By encouraging my deep interest in animals and nature, my parents let me grow into a highly curious individual who was never bored—I was fascinated by so many different things. I always had something interesting to do—always had a major project out there waiting to be worked on—like the cabin (and like this book!).

The lakefront property and the small cabin on it were in a state of disrepair and required quite a bit of fixing up on weekends—a great distraction for me as my first year of being cancer-free approached. At night we'd put bread, corn, and apples out on the large lawn of wild grass to watch the deer, raccoons, gray foxes, skunks, armadillos, and possums come to feed at twilight.

The nearest general store to get food was in the incredibly tiny town of Olustee, the site of a tide-turning Civil War battle that is reenacted there every year. Besides that historical site, the only thing in the town of Olustee is that little general store.

On our heavily forested five-acre plot, we had all sorts of large wild animals wandering through. The most notable of these was the endangered Florida cougar, whose large tracks often crossed the sand driveway that led up to our cabin. Some of these big cats had radio transmitter collars on them, put there by scientists studying the extent of this endangered predator's natural range.

But there are also black bears, wild boar, white-tailed deer, bobcats—you name it, Osceola National Forest has it—plus enormous alligators, snapping turtles, canebrake rattlesnakes, and water moccasins. And let's not forget the small red, yellow, and black banded coral snake, easily recognized as deadly compared to similar-colored harmless snakes by using the little backwoods ditty, "Red and yeller kills a feller."

When I would ask my friends if they wanted to go swimming with me in the large lake the cabin looked out over, I would rarely get takers. But I would never get takers at night. That's when the really big gators were out trolling for trouble.

Peggy and I spent a lot of time fixing up the cabin, painting it inside and out, building a deck and a screened-in porch. We even put in an outdoor shower for washing under the stars, the thunderous sound of the bullfrogs and bellowing alligators warming up our human spirit. Likewise, it must have warmed the Native Americans who hunted these forests long ago when they were ruled by Chief Osceola, the legendary Indian warrior and now the namesake of this vast region comprised of pine forests and cypress swamps.

Rocky made a couple of trips up to the cabin on weekends with Peggy and me and the kids, but he never seemed to enjoy car rides like Peanut, our Yorkie, does. So, we doubled up his food and water and gave him a break from us on a lot of Saturday nights. He always appeared a little bit better rested when we'd get back to our Fleming Island home late on Sunday afternoons.

Traveling to and fixing up the cabin deep into the woods—and getting some quality rest and quiet time—always helped buoy my spirits. This was especially true when Peggy, Brian, Christie, and I would take our telescope out late at night and sit it on the cabin's front deck to study the planets in the dark forest sky, without any of the light pollution now common in the night sky surrounding cities and suburbs. In the Osceola National Forest the night sky was filled with one hundred times the stars we could see from our home outside Jacksonville. It was magnificent. If the countless trillions of stars in the sky are all similar to the sun we orbit, how many of them have a planet like earth circling them at a distance not too hot for life and not too cold for it either?

Scientists now believe one of the stars in the Big Dipper has a solar system with planets in orbits around it just like earth's trajectory around the sun. It's certainly something to think about next time you see the Big Dipper. If there is another planet like earth out there, is there another Bill Goss out there with a pet flying squirrel named Rocky? I kind of doubt it.

The sky—boy, do I ever love gazing up at the sky. But, even more so, I love gazing down at Mother Earth from high above. I was no longer flying military planes, but I occasionally got to fly airplanes that my friends owned.

One of them, Pat Coyle, had a sixty-year-old amphibious plane called a Sea-Bee, which can land on water or land. We were soon talking about flying it to Osceola National Forest, and landing it in Ocean Pond, the large wilderness lake our cabin was on.

But before we were able to do that, Pat and I were flying down the St. Johns River, right past our house. Suddenly the engine started to falter. Since it had only one engine and the weather was getting kind of stormy and rough, we decided it would be smart to do a water landing on Doctor's Lake, just a few miles from where Peggy and I live. Just as we were about to touch down, the engine quit and we landed on the center of the large lake. Eventually we got the attention of some people on a houseboat who offered to tow us to Pat's house about a mile away. It must have been an odd sight—a house towing a plane across a lake to another house. I'm glad we put that old bird down when we did. I'd had it with plane crashes.

Pat wasn't so lucky with that old amphibious plane. But then again, maybe he was damn lucky. Shortly after our misadventure flying together, Pat was flying the Sea-Bee alone over central Florida and the engine blew up. He miraculously did a successful dead-stick crash landing in a cow pasture. But when he got out of his plane to kiss the ground in gratitude, suddenly, from out of nowhere, a huge bull in a full high-speed charge appeared and tried to gore him to death. Pat had to jump onto his plane's left wing to avoid almost getting killed for a second time in only just a few minutes. According to my good buddy Pat, who works full-time as a U.S. Customs pilot, this is a certified no-bull story.

I prefer flying Pat's V-tail Bonanza with retractable gear. It's old too, but it's much faster and more reliable than the Sea-Bee. Its only flaw is it doesn't land on water, something I consider a particularly handy feature when flying over northeastern Florida.

Thankfully, time moved on without the cancer recurring, but Peggy and I still had several scares, particularly when lymph nodes in my armpits seemed to become larger and more pronounced. This can be a very bad indicator of the way things are evolving for a malignant melanoma survivor, because this disease typically metastasizes within the lymphatic system. Many cancer survivors, very aware of this fact, soap up their underarms when they shower and feel around with their fingers, carefully checking for any lumps or other abnormalities. I know I do. And if I feel anything, it's right to the doctor, because, without a doubt, when dealing with cancer, the earlier, the better.

Usually a swollen lymph node is caused by an infection from a cold or flu or even a cut, but cancer survivors have to be extra cautious. A good general rule for anyone is this: If a possible swollen lymph node or lump under the skin sticks around for more than a few days or feels like it's growing bigger, you should see a doctor immediately.

Luckily, in my case, the lumps in my armpits (after several needle biopsies) were revealed to be either slightly enlarged lymph nodes from a minor infection or unusually small hard muscles from doing a lot of fingertip push-ups.

One of the most valuable set of rules about skin cancer, and particularly malignant melanoma, has been promoted by the National Cancer Institute, the American Cancer Society, and the American Melanoma Foundation. It pertains to the moles and unusual bumps and marks we sometimes find on our skin. I call it simply the ABCDE-and-I rule. It is very useful to use as a memory aid in determining whether a mole on the skin is potentially deadly or not.

A is for Asymmetry. Is the mole perfectly round or is one half distinctly different than the other half? If it is, you should have a dermatologist look at it.

B is for Border. Is the mole's border very distinct or is it diffused or ragged-looking? If the border is not distinct or is ragged, you should have a dermatologist take a look at it.

C is for Color. Is your mole's color evenly distributed or is the color or shading uneven? If it is uneven, schedule an appoint with your dermatologist.

D is for Diameter. Is the mole's diameter greater than that of a pencil eraser? If so, call your dermatologist.

E is for Elevated. This is kind of new to the rules. Is the mole perfectly smooth to the touch like the surrounding skin or can you feel something—even if it is only a tiny something—underneath the mole? If you can feel the mole is elevated, visit your dermatologist.

And last is I. I is my own idea. I is for Itch. I learned this from personal experience and then I read about it later as sometimes being a symptom of malignant melanoma. Does your mole itch? Basal cell carcinomas and squamous cell carcinomas, the two most common forms of skin cancer, normally do not itch. But malignant melanoma, the rarest and deadliest form of skin cancer, often does itch, and this can be a dead giveaway to a serious problem lurking within your mole.

My left ear—which did not have a mole on it, just a small bump beneath perfectly clear skin—itched like crazy. It was one of the biggest reasons why I continued to pester the Navy flight surgeon into removing it from my ear. Thank God she sent it to the pathology laboratory.

So there you have it: ABCDE and I. Asymmetric, Border, Color, Diameter, Elevated, and Itch. Any one of these things should give you a reason to have a dermatologist look at your skin. A mole with several of these traits should get the attention of a dermatologist immediately.

Former President Reagan's first daughter, Maureen, died of malignant melanoma. When it first started out as a spot on the back of her left thigh, five years earlier, Maureen was not too concerned. But she stated that when it started looking "gushy," she knew it was time to see a doctor. But it was already too late. After a year of surgical procedures and treatment with interferon to boost her immune system, which left her feeling sick, as with a bad flu, Maureen was hopeful.

But four years later the melanoma was back and within a few months it had spread to her liver, right arm, her groin, and one of her ribs. Not long afterward, it invaded her brain, and within a few months she was dead. While she waged her personal battle against cancer, she continued to crusade against it publicly as well. She was completely convinced that, with early detection and appropriate treatment due to greater public awareness, the skin cancer epidemic could be stopped.

It is not an exaggeration that it is reaching epidemic proportions. This year over one million Americans will be diagnosed with skin cancer. Approximately 75 percent will be basal cell, 20 percent will be squamous cell, and only 5 percent will be malignant melanoma.

Melanoma, the least common skin cancer but by far the deadliest, strikes twice as many people now as it did only thirty years ago. It is now one of the most common cancers in people between the ages of twenty-five and twenty-nine, when all other cancers are a rarity.

I was almost thirty-nine when I was diagnosed, and waiting for that first year to pass cancer-free was sometimes a bit tedious. But finally the big day arrived. A fortieth-birthday party that was welcomed by me with open arms. Me, the happy—deliriously happy—old fart. Forty years young. This birthday was a milestone, with far greater meaning than the typical "over the hump" party, which I think should have a great deal of meaning anyway. I had gotten to my fortieth without a cancer recurrence—and for me and my family and friends, that was huge. Really huge.

Peggy and I had a blowout birthday party at the River House, just about five miles up the river from our house. The River House is located in the clubhouse of the ancient golf course Margaret Seton Fleming helped create over one hundred years ago. When someone bought the historic Fleming family estate and decided to turn the old nine-hole golf course into a housing development, which is now called Hibernia Links, they planned on leveling the clubhouse to the ground. Someone came up with the bright idea of saving the rustic clubhouse by putting it on a giant barge and floating it five miles up the St. Johns River and placing it beside the beautiful old mansion of the Massey family, one of the founders of the Colgate Palmolive Company. The mansion, no longer a family home, is a country club called Club Continental and also serves as a unique and upscale bed-and-breakfast.

My fortieth birthday party began on the back deck of the River House on one of the widest parts of the St. Johns River, but I have no idea where it ended. I'm sure the manatee and alligators stuck their heads out of the water to see what all of the ruckus was about.

It was a wonderful time. Friends and family traveled in from all over the country. Old Navy pilot buddies appeared from out of nowhere (whenever there is a cold keg of beer being tapped, this is not an unlikely phenomenon). Some of the doctors and nurses who had worked on me over the past year showed up with big smiles on their faces.

Having broken through the one year cancer-free milestone,

I felt forty years young, though so much wiser than just one year before. I could now start measuring my remaining life in years instead of days.

I didn't resent turning forty at all. Not one bit. Cancer can put a whole new spin on things.

8

My Left Ear: The Reconstruction of Bill Goss

*T*he one-year cancer-free mark. What a milestone! Not only was I eternally grateful, but it meant the reconstruction of my left ear could get started, under the hands of naval doctor Eric Weiss, an extremely talented thirty-something plastic surgeon.

I imagine Rocky, especially from his morning perch on top of my head, was sick and tired of peering down at an ear that looked like the unfortunate result of a boxing match with Mike Tyson. Personally, I don't know what I would have done if someone had bitten off a piece of my ear during a World Heavyweight title bout, especially after it was done a second time in the same fight, but Evander Holyfield took it like a real gentleman. Tyson should have been disbarred from professional boxing for life. Sometimes when we use the expression "they behaved like animals," we're not being fair to our four-footed friends.

But regardless of what Rocky was thinking, I too wanted to start looking normal again. I wanted to do something to stop strangers from staring at me in public. I wanted a matching set of ears. Who wouldn't?

This didn't seem like a very tall order, but according to plastic surgeons, it was. Ears are one of the most difficult parts of the body to reconstruct.

The reconstruction appeared to go well at first. Dr. Weiss shaved a large piece of skin off my left leg to use for grafting, and removed one of my ribs so that he could harvest cartilage from it to give my ear some internal structure, like the skeleton does for the entire body. Like a master furniture maker, but instead using living skin and bones, scalpels and scissors, needles and thread, Dr. Weiss did his magic and then tightly wrapped my head and ear in a pressure dressing to hold the whole thing together as it healed. He also rigged a test tube to the side of my head to catch any drainage from the reconstruction site. This quickly filled with blood and by the time I got home from the hospital, my son, Brian, took a look at me, and especially at the red-filled test tube dangling from the pressure dressing over my left ear like a humming-bird feeder.

"You better not go outside, Daddy," he said. "I don't want you to get pecked to death by hummingbirds."

A few weeks later, with great expectations—mine—Dr. Weiss removed the pressure dressing and examined my new ear.

"Bill, this is bad," he stated with disappointment. His wonderful craftsmanship had been in vain. My new ear was rotting, not healing. The skin graft had not taken. And if something wasn't done rather quickly, the risk of getting a dangerous infection was very high.

Dr. Weiss explained that the graft had likely failed because the layer of skin he had harvested from my thigh was too thin. It would not allow an adequate supply of oxygenated blood from the rest of my body to readily circulate in and out of my left ear.

"We'll start over again first thing tomorrow morning, Bill. This time we'll have to get a much thicker piece of skin for the graft."

"From where?" I responded rather sheepishly.

He smiled. "I think you already know."

Early the following morning in the operating room, the whole thing started all over again, but this time, I chose a local anesthesia rather than go under a general. I figured if Dr. Weiss and his surgical team were going to harvest a thick piece of skin from my groin to use to rebuild my left ear, I wanted to be awake and alert, to hear what was going on. I didn't want them to make any mistakes while they were down there, if you know what I mean.

I studied self-hypnosis under one of the great masters, Dr. Harry Aaron, while I was at Rutgers. I put what Dr. Aaron had taught me to good use on my second ear-reconstruction operation. Dr. Weiss had warned me that if I made any sounds or sudden movements because I was feeling pain while he worked on me, it would really tick him off and he might end up cutting off more than he—or I—had bargained for. Yikes. "Yeah, sure, Doc. I'll be still. I promise."

And still I was, self-hypnotized, but completely conscious and aware throughout the entire operation, listening to the highly entertaining banter of the doctors and nurses, led by Dr. Weiss, as they cut off and stitched on stuff I would have preferred to stay in the place where it was when I was born.

One of the main reasons I wanted to try self-hypnosis during the reconstructive surgery was that the first attempt at rebuilding my left ear may have been hindered by the presence of general anesthesia in my blood. This time, I hoped, using self-hypnosis and a local anesthesia would help to provide a higher quality of blood to the graft site immediately. I was also hoping this would be a big help in the healing process, because if this reconstructive surgery didn't work, I probably would not be able to persuade the hospital to schedule me for another one. So I was looking at this as my last chance to get a new left ear. And I wanted it bad.

Rocky was banned from his favorite perch on my head over the next few weeks. If Dr. Weiss discovered that a nonsterile flying squirrel (sorry, Rocky) was climbing all over my medical wraps, he'd have every right to be annoyed with me. I absolutely could not afford to run the risk of getting an infected skin graft. I could lose the little bit of ear I had left. And an infection that close to your brain is never a good thing.

So again, with great anticipation, a few weeks later, Dr. Weiss took off my pressure dressing to look at his second attempt at giving me a new ear. Voilà! My new and improved ear was hanging tight. It had properly scabbed up. The skin was pink, not black. This ear was here to stay.

Dr. Weiss was pleased too, but he jokingly cautioned me not to be overly optimistic.

"Bill, since the skin graft came from your groin, you'll probably have to shave your left ear every couple of days," he said. Then he added with a broad grin, "And you can imagine what's going to happen to your ear when your wife kisses you good night."

9

The Luckiest Unlucky Man Alive

A t about eighteen months of age, Rocky was full-grown now, at a fighting weight of about three ounces. I didn't notice that extra weight he had put on since Rocky had fallen from the sky and into our lives. Well, maybe he was leaving a slightly wider part in my hair.

My retirement from the Navy became official. It gave me quite a bit to think about, my first career having gone by seemingly in the blink of an eye. How could it have gone by so fast? Had it been a waste of time? How much real life value and experience had occurred in those twenty years? Good question, and worth pondering. It turned out there had been quite a lot of value over that span of time. And there was quite a lot to reflect upon.

Besides allowing me the honor of serving in the U.S. Armed

Forces in defense of the United States of America, the Navy provided me with opportunities to do and see so many incredible things that, in retrospect, I think I would have done it for free. Especially true for someone still a teenager when he signed up, a wide-eyed nineteen-year-old New Jersey garbage man and New York Yankees parking lot attendant who was dying to travel around the world but without any funds to do such a grandiose thing. A basically regular kid with a pretty good sense of values and a sense of who he was, a guy who had been self-sufficient and independent for quite some time, due to the truckloads of self-reliance bestowed on him by his parents.

Twenty years. From a robust, unmarried, enlisted teenager without a college degree, to a married military officer and Navy pilot, the father of twins, with an MBA and an Airline Transport Pilot (ATP) rating—and a history of cancer. A lot of stuff had happened in that period of time.

I guess I would be remiss if I didn't do a quick review of my two decades in the Navy. Without it, you really wouldn't have a very good idea of who I was or what I had been through to turn into the person I am now.

In every foreign country I lived in or visited while in the Navy, often armed with a handful of brochures my travel-agent mom sent to me from the agency she worked at in Short Hills, New Jersey, I visited the nontourist communities and, when possible, the wilds of every locale imaginable, with the goal to soak up as much local color and flora and fauna as was possible in the time I had available. When visiting a foreign country, I didn't sleep. I learned about the culture. I explored as much as possible.

So, upon my medical retirement from the military at age thirty-nine, I put down on paper a quick review of what I had done and where I had been the last twenty years, along with a few internationally historical milestones. What follows is what I came up with.

After two semesters as a long-haired student at the University of Arizona and almost dying in a cave-in while setting up dynamite five thousand feet underground in a copper mine I was working in to pay for college, I drove my old Volvo back home and enlisted in the United States Navy in Newark, New Jersey.

I attended boot camp in Orlando, Florida; Mine Warfare Training in Charleston, South Carolina; then the fall of Saigon, Vietnam, occurred.

Then I served as an Underwater Weapons Specialist in Long Beach, California; worked on board the aircraft carrier USS *Ranger* in the Pacific Ocean; worked for the admiral in charge of all U.S. Navy Mine Warfare Operations headquartered in Charleston, South Carolina. Next, I was transferred overseas and I lived and worked in Italy and Scotland. I visited Malta, Germany, England, and Wales.

Then I started getting serious with Peggy, a waitress working her way through college, after being introduced to her by my best buddy, Jeff Marcketta, one year earlier.

After getting an honorable discharge from the Navy, I used the G.I. Bill to attend Rutgers University in New Jersey. I stayed in the Navy Reserve while at Rutgers and built underwater bombs as a "weekend warrior" at the nearby Earle Naval Weapon Station. I boxed light-heavyweight division in the New Jersey Golden Gloves in Newark, New Jersey; graduated Rutgers with a degree in business and economics; completed the sixteen-week "Officer and a Gentleman" Naval Aviation Officer Training Program in Pensacola, Florida, and received my commission as an ensign in the United States Navy.

Peggy and I eloped a few days later. We were married by the justice of the peace in Pensacola, then we jumped into my old Volvo 122S and drove to our next duty station, in Corpus Christi, Texas, where I started Navy Pilot Training, flying the 1,425-horsepower T-28 Trojan as my first airplane. Eighteen months later I earned the highly coveted Navy Pilot Wings of Gold.

Peggy and I traveled through northern Mexico, then we were transferred to advanced flight training in Jacksonville, Florida. There I was trained to pilot the P-3 Orion, an aircraft designed to spy on, track, and, if ordered to do so, attack and blow up any submerged Soviet submarine that had its long-range nuclear missiles targeting the cities bordering the eastern seaboard of the United States.

Peggy and I then bought and moved into our first home, in Bath, Maine; I went on six-month deployments to Bermuda, Italy, Spain, with classified flight missions off the coast of Libya, over Antarctica, and I made trips to the countries of Iceland, Greenland, Canada, France, Germany, Barbados, Gibraltar, and parts of North Africa. From the Italian island of Sardinia, I traveled down to twelve hundred feet beneath the surface of the Mediterranean during the sea trials of the nuclear submarine USS *Whale*. Later, I survived a major crash landing in a P-3 Orion on a runway at the naval air station in Rota, Spain.

I was then transferred back to Texas to be an advanced instructor pilot of students in multi-engine aircraft. Peggy and I bought our second home. I won the Navy League Officer of the Year Award. I got the opportunity to fly T-2 Buckeye jets and TA-4 Skyhawk jets on and off the aircraft carrier USS *Lexington*, plus I got to fly a variety of helicopters and other aircraft. I also flew my own ultralight aircraft, a Pterodactyl, on and off the beach on Padre Island, where we lived.

The crowning achievement of our life together, Peggy and I were blessed with the birth of our twins, Christie and Brian, beautiful and healthy, with none of the birth complications occasionally associated with having twins.

I finally earned an MBA after five years of night school. I received the Navy Pilot Writer of the Year Award and the Navy Flight Instructor of the Quarter Award.

My next transfer was to San Diego for a few months of Ship Navigation School, then right up to the San Francisco Bay Area to be the assistant navigator of one of the newest nuclear aircraft carriers, the USS *Carl Vinson*. I worked on the bridge of the ship directly for the captain and the navigator. I navigated the ship under the Oakland Bay Bridge, then under the Golden Gate out to Pearl Harbor, Hawaii, throughout the Alaskan Aleutian Islands, Japan, Korea, the Philippines, conducting extensive twenty-four-hour flight operations throughout the Pacific while transiting between these various countries. I qualified as an Officer of the Deck of the ship while it was under way.

When the giant earthquake struck San Francisco, smacking Peggy and the kids to the ground, I was on the other side of the world, on the USS *Carl Vinson*, completely miserable along with six thousand other sailors. Stuck off the coast of Pusan, Korea, we were unable to contact our families to see if they survived. Later we learned that the top deck of the Oakland Bay Bridge collapsed on a commuter van, killing the wife of one of our officers. He was flown off the ship later that day to attend her funeral.

I was awarded the Navy Commendation Medal for my work on the ship, then was transferred to Jacksonville, Florida, to fly the P-3 Orion spy plane again. I was struck by a speeding, out-of-control 1965 Ford Fairlane and knocked forty-five feet through the air. I checked out of the hospital after three days, and not long afterward, I piloted a P-3 Orion to Holland. Not long after that, I started flying missions out of Iceland and France; the Soviet Union fell; the Cold War ended; I got a job working for the admiral responsible for the major naval installations in the southeastern United States; I broke the sound-barrier with a friend of mine in a Navy F-18 Hornet. Then I was diagnosed with cancer, had twelve hours of radical cancer surgery, and retired.

I felt compelled to review the high and low points of my twenty years in the military to illustrate to young men and women seeking travel, adventure, one-of-a-kind training opportunities, and rich life experiences, and who have the desire to serve their country, that such an opportunity still exists in the Navy and the other branches of the Armed Services and National Guard. Though I'm biased, like John F. Kennedy when he said, "Any man who may be asked what he did to make his life worthwhile, I think can respond with a good deal of pride and satisfaction: 'I served in the United States Navy.' "

I learned at an early age that if you want something, you go for it, and the younger you are when you get started, the more fulfilled your life is likely to be. And hopefully it will be such a rich life that you will always want to continue to move forward toward your dreams, unafraid of the struggles and challenges that lay ahead of you, with greater wisdom, resolve—and a sense of humor—than ever before.

The most important thing I wanted to do after retirement was to be the best damn father, husband, son, sibling, and friend to those nearest and dearest to me. Retirement. Damn.

Finally I could slow things down a notch or two and start smelling the roses a little bit more. Finally, Peggy and I would be able to determine our own schedules.

My calendar opened up enough to allow me to start saying yes to requests to be a guest speaker at local schools, clubs, associations, and corporations, sometimes accompanied by the inimitable Rocky.

It was the first time I took the Rock with me on one of these engagements that I realized how powerful a bond had developed between the Rockster and myself. In front of twenty-five nine-year-olds, Rocky jumped from his open cage door up onto my leg. Then, much to the delight of the entire classroom, he shot up my leg and planted a big kiss right on my lips. Continuing up to the top of my head like a bullet, he then perched in my hair like it was a bird's nest, eating a pecan while surveying the joyfully laughing children below, feeling safe, high up in his squirreldom.

It was an adorable and captivating display of mutual love and affection between a somewhat macho 6-foot, 190-pound Navy pilot and a tiny 6-inch, 3-ounce flying squirrel. And, even though Rocky was nocturnal and normally slept throughout the day, the Rockster demonstrated a willingness to wake right up and put on a show for the audience. In front of a crowd he was far more animated in personality—like the fictitious Rocky the Flying Squirrel—than anyone would ever have expected.

I was his Bullwinkle—better yet, his Billwinkle.

Since I was a kid, I'd been asked to bring animals to school auditoriums to share with people of all ages how wonderful a relationship can exist between humans and animals. This was particularly true with a group of animals that most people both detest and are unfamiliar with—reptiles and amphibians.

Often, when I brought a snake or two out to show people, the audience's fascination was extreme. Remarkably, within moments, I would have people who had once harbored a deadly fear of snakes excitedly touching, then holding a beautiful red rat snake or king snake, local species relatively common in the people's own backyards. And the snakes would enjoy their newfound friends as much as the people holding them, because snakes appear to like being cradled in our warm hands. Snakes are cold-blooded, so they seek out warmth, and the 98.6 degrees of the human body is certainly better than the 72 degrees of your typical school auditorium.

The thing most striking to people formerly afraid of snakes is that they thought snakes were deadly, dirty, and slimy. Instead, they learn to their delight that most snakes are completely harmless and have clean, dry skin that is silky smooth. Most snakes truly have a wonderful feel. They're actually a pleasure to touch. And most are helpful, not harmful.

Many of us have very powerful fears simply due to being conditioned that way because of a bad childhood experience, or due to a lack of education or understanding. Doing a few of these snake-education programs showed me how quickly even the most imbedded and terrifying fears can fly right out the window—permanently—if the fear-related issues are handled properly.

With these reptile programs, there was always a sense of learning and fascination. But with a Rocky show, it was different. Audiences were blown away by the adorableness of it all. They could immediately relate with the loving bond that had developed between Rocky and me. No education or quest for greater understanding was necessary. When these kids went home after meeting Rocky and me, they probably reinforced the special relationships they had with their own dogs, cats, rabbits, or birds. Because we are distracted by so many different things, we can inadvertently take even our most valuable relationships for granted, not only among family members and friends, but even with the relationship we have with our pets.

Well, at Paterson Elementary School anyway, evidently I'd left a favorable enough impression with my last Rocky the Flying Squirrel visit that Fred Fedorowich, the principal, asked me to give the sixth-graders a motivational talk at their graduation ceremony. This time he wanted me without Rocky, and he asked me to give some kind of talk that would help the kids build up their confidence and reduce their fears before they entered the complex world of raging hormones and junior high school.

Fred had read a copy of my first book and liked the inspiration and motivation within its pages, particularly with regards to perseverance. Even though I've told parents not to let their kids read *The Luckiest Unlucky Man Alive* until they themselves had first read it (because I wrote the book strictly for adults), Fred still thought the overall theme of the Five Fs of Fulfillment was terrific for kids: Family, Friends, Faith, Focus, and Fun. Even as kids, one of our primary goals is to feel fulfilled.

Mr. Fedorowich also read a three-page story I wrote that had been published in *Chicken Soup for the Pet Lover's Soul*, a book that ended up on *The New York Times* best-seller list. Coauthored by Jack Canfield, Mark Victor Hansen, world-renowned veterinarian Dr. Marty Becker, and Carol Kline, it's a wonderful collection of stories about pets as teachers, healers, heroes, and friends.

My book, *The Luckiest Unlucky Man Alive*, also contained a

small story about Rocky. After my book and *Chicken Soup for the Pet Lover's Soul* were published, I started getting calls from newspaper and television reporters from all over the world. My *Chicken Soup for the Pet Lover's Soul* story was used in China as an instructional aid to teach English. Soon, my life, Peggy's life, Brian and Christie's lives—and Rocky's life— would never be the same.

The first phone call came from a producer of *The 700 Club*, who invited me to be a guest on their internationally broadcast television show. I accepted, they sent me a plane ticket, and I flew up to their Virginia Beach campus and broadcasting studios, where I was interviewed on live television by Pat Robertson's son, Gordon. It was fun, and I guess some viewers found my story inspirational because, a few days later, I started receiving a lot of nice letters from viewers all over the world.

The next call came from the internationally broadcast TV news magazine show *Extra*, based in Los Angeles. They ended up sending a producer, cameraman, and sound person to our home on Fleming Island for a day. This too was fun, and the *Extra* crew got Peggy, Christie, and Brian involved in a lot of the shoots. It ended up being a beautifully produced piece that was broadcast three times over the next year. Then came a German show called *Satellite One*, which is broadcast throughout Europe and the Mediterranean, followed by my infamous radio interview with Howard Stern, the multi-million-dollar megamouth, an interview that ended up being quite lengthy and yet still went surprisingly well. It was a sensationally funny interview. I still think Howard Stern's a jerk and a pig, but, in his own way, a goofy, likable kind of jerk and pig. Compared to so many other guests he's had on his show, even some major celebrities, Howard treated me like a prince. He asked me a ton of questions, mostly about all the lucky and unlucky experiences I'd been through. He and his sidekick, Robin, seemed fascinated by my many brushes with death. He included sound effects in the background as I told some of these stories on the air. I don't think Howard's ever really been physically in harm's way. He's never been a risk taker with his body, only with his mouth. At least that's the way I interpreted it when he said to me, "This is the stuff I'm interested in, Bill, because I've never had anything like this happen to me." I almost felt sorry for him. He should definitely get out and have more adventures in the great outdoors.

After I had been invited to be a guest on Howard's show, I asked one of my more devout friends, Rudy Ruettiger, if I should accept the invitation, because I had been planning to turn Howard down.

"Yes, absolutely, go on his show!" Rudy said, after he had thought about it for a moment.

"Why would you advise me to go on his show, Rudy?" I asked, incredulous.

"Because when you're telling your story on a show like *The 700 Club*, you're inspiring a unique group of people who are turning the show on just to be inspired. Their goal is to be inspired. But on Howard's show, Bill, you'll be talking to a completely different group of people. And they're real unique, too! These people aren't listening to Howard to be inspired, but to be shocked and entertained. But your story will inspire them anyway. You'll be helping a whole new group of people. Go on his show—I think you'll do awesome, Bill!" Rudy was right. The interview went exceptionally well. It's wonderful to count Rudy among my very close friends.

My Howard Stern radio interview was followed by many other radio interviews across the United States, many of them patched in over the phone from our home in Florida. Some of these interviews were only five minutes long while others were over an hour. Surprisingly, it was some of the biggest radio hosts who had me on the air for the longest. Howard, knowing I wasn't particularly a fan of his, concluded his lengthy interview with this remark about me: "Any guy who survived all that and also served his country, if you want to go out and bad-mouth me, I say go ahead, what the hell."

I also did radio interviews in Canada, Italy, Australia, New Zealand, and even one in Malaysia. Easily 50 percent of the message I got out to people on these shows, even on Howard Stern, was about the essential need for the earliest possible detection of cancer, especially malignant melanoma. And I always try to review the ABCDE-and-I rule about skin cancer with my audience so that people immediately have something with which to evaluate any questionable moles on their bodies.

Two other major radio celebrities who interviewed me live on the air and who were personally fascinated and concerned about cancer and particularly malignant melanoma were Rick Dees, the Los Angeles–based disc jockey who wrote and sang the wacky tune "Disco Duck," and Ted Nugent, also known as the Motor City Madman of Detroit. Famous for the rock anthem "Cat Scratch Fever," Ted Nugent sold more rock albums in the eighties than just about anyone else in the world.

I did a live interview with Rick Dees from my home phone in Florida. Originally from Jacksonville, Dees had a lot of fun with that secret little bit of information. He made so many insightful remarks about the tiniest details of Jacksonville that

I was stunned by the research he must have conducted prior to our interview. I told him so on the air. When he came clean and told me that he was a native of Jacksonville, I had a pretty good laugh.

After the interview he invited me out to do a live radio interview in his spectacular office suite in Los Angeles, with his sidekick, the former *Playboy* model Ellen K. I went out there and again discussed skin cancer in detail to his huge radio audience during morning drive time to work. After talking about cancer, Rick and I did his famous Battle of the Sexes game. It was a series of questions from Rick and Ellen directed at me and a female phone-in caller. I won the Battle of the Sexes with this question from Ellen K: "Bill, how many milligrams per day does the average woman require of calcium . . . one thousand milligrams, fifteen hundred milligrams, or twenty five hundred?" I guessed the correct answer—fifteen hundred milligrams—so I won the Battle of the Sexes that day for the guys. I told you I was lucky. It was interesting how a disc jockey like Rick Dees was, in his own way, using the radio airwaves to help people learn more about their health and their bodies.

During the Motor City Madman's radio interview with me, Ted Nugent was particularly interested in having a discussion about cancer. It turned out that Ted's mother, a woman whom he adored, had died after a very courageous battle with breast cancer.

Not long afterward, I got a call from my close friend Bill Beck, out in Montana. I could tell something was wrong. Seriously wrong.

Bill had grown up in the house that backed up to ours in Millburn, New Jersey. Four years older than I, Bill was an amazing athlete, particularly in track and field, where he broke the state record in the 880-yard run. He was also a wildlife and wilderness fanatic. In many ways, he became my mentor in the ways of wild animals and the great outdoors.

Bill went out west for college and then started running raft trips out of Jackson Hole, Wyoming. A few years later, with another very close friend of mine, Dr. Allan Speidell, they acquired a spectacular piece of mountain wilderness property called Bear Creek Ranch at the base of Glacier National Park in northwestern Montana. After running this combination hunting lodge and dude ranch for ten years, Bill married a great lady named Lora. They began a family together, raising two handsome young sons.

Bill's call to me was bad news. His wife, Lora, had battled breast cancer a few years earlier and it had suddenly returned with a vengeance. She was extremely sick and completely bedridden in the local hospital. I told Bill that if he wanted me to, I would come out to help him in any way I could. He accepted.

Montana is God's country. At Bear Creek Ranch, the back-range view of Glacier National Park and the Bob Marshall Wilderness Complex is simply breathtaking. You can often spot grizzly bears—not black bears, but true grizzlies—clearly visible on the nearby mountain slope digging for ground squirrels. Enormous in size, easily North America's most powerful carnivore, it's hard to put into words what the sight of one of these spectacular animals in the wild does to the soul in terms of reminding us of the awe-inspiring power of nature in all her true majesty.

Bill stayed by Lora's hospital bedside as she was dosed up with enormous amounts of morphine to kill the pain from the tumors that had spread to her bones. Seeing Bill and his sons by Lora's side, day after day, week after week, was one of the more touching and moving things I've ever witnessed. I watched each day as poor Lora became completely comatose and shrank to less than half her normal weight. I watched Bill and their boys—and Lora's father and sister—suffer in terrible silence along with beautiful Lora. And I truly came to understand just how horrible a disease breast cancer can be. Lora died just a few weeks short of her forty-fifth birthday. Mothers, especially with those young children, should not be dying of cancer. But it often takes efforts at the grass-roots level to change things.

And so Bill, intuitively knowing this and a natural-born activist of sorts, started the Lora Beck Memorial Foundation. In its first year, it raised over one million dollars to fund the development of a new hospital so the people in his community could have better access to early cancer detection technologies and other modern procedures. He did this in the hopes that other women with young children at home would not be struck down in the prime of their lives.

Looking out onto the most amazing mountain vistas in North America, East Glacier Lodge was described in a guidebook as "the world's largest log cabin." Bill asked me to speak there at one of his earliest fundraising events for the Lora Beck Memorial Foundation. Once you see the enormous tree trunks holding the massive roof in place, you will understand the magnitude of this understatement. What a magnificent place to hold a fundraiser in honor of Lora and her love of the wilderness.

Bill's resolve to have Lora's memory live on in such a meaningful and lasting way is, to me, a noble and beautiful thing, especially in this unique and exquisite corner of wild America.

When Ted Nugent learned that Lora's breast cancer had

spread to her bones, like it had with his own mother years earlier, he made several inspiring phone calls to Bill, who remained steadfast at Lora's side throughout the several-month ordeal.

Lora Beck had been an outdoor track star and a huge lover of Mother Nature, the wilderness, and her family and friends. After her painful struggle was finally over and she passed on, Bill Beck received a touching e-mail with just these seven words: "Bill, in the wind, Lora's still alive." It was signed "Your BBT." It took Bill and me just a moment to figure out who that e-mail came from— "Your Blood Brother Ted."

After the radio interview with Ted Nugent where he and I had a detailed discussion about cancer, he invited me to be his guest when he opened the House of Blues in Orlando. It was fun. On stage he is beyond wild with a guitar, truly earning his nickname, the Motor City Madman. But, remarkably, as soon as he leaves the stage, he instantly turns off the rock-star persona and simply becomes a happily married guy who adores his wife and kids. Ted is also a major bow-hunting, wildlife, and wilderness activist, and he adores his own pet dogs and cats.

Ted's an extremist in a very patriotic American sense of the word. He's an extreme individual—and an extreme American. Once you meet him, he's hard not to like—just as long as you don't judge who he is from his stage performance alone.

Ted summed up my appearance on his show that morning with this typically extreme remark to all of surrounding Detroit, live, on the air:

"I'm definitely moved by Bill Goss's luck, and I'm definitely moved by his book *The Luckiest Unlucky Man Alive* and the photos within it. I'm definitely moved that you would be on my radio show, and I'm moved by the beauty and stimuli of your wife. You're a true Nugent warrior, Bill Goss—and I salute you!"

With the many radio interviews I did across the country, besides trying to educate people about cancer in a way that was captivating and entertaining, I would try to talk about my Five Fs of Fulfillment: Family, Friends, Faith, Focus, and Fun. I quickly learned that if you aren't stimulating on the radio, if you are a downer, the morning-drive time listeners will turn to another station in about three seconds, and the radio interviewer-hosts will lose their ratings.

So, before the listeners tune you out, the hosts find a way to get rid of you quickly. Conversely, if you are really fascinating and lively, the interviewers will keep you on the air projecting your message for much longer than they had originally planned. In a nutshell, on the radio, especially with the morning drive-time shows, you must quickly captivate the audience with your stories and at the same time boost the hosts' egos (which are often enormous) or you will be gone in sixty seconds.

On longer shows, I would usually find a way to talk about how having little Rocky fall out of the sky and into my life was an integral part of the reason I was not only surviving cancer, I was thriving in the very face of it. And how having Rocky living in our kitchen was a joy to the entire Goss household, even our dog, Peanut. How, if you don't have joy in your home, you'd better find a way to get some in there quick, because without any joy, it's not going to be a home for long. And how sometimes the tiniest of animals, no bigger than a walnut—like a tiny baby flying squirrel—is just what you need to bring joy back into your home, your life, and the lives of your loved ones.

Internationally, the *London Sun* did a full-page story about some of the challenges I had been through. Their big headline read, MR. LUCKY. "This man survived a plane crash, car smash, shooting, mining disaster, explosive blast and cancer." It ended up generating a lot of calls from newspapers and television shows all over Europe.

One German newspaper had this headline: BILL GOSS SPRANG DEM SICHEREN TOD SHON 30MAL VON DER SCHIPPE. My father translated it to English to mean something like "Bill Goss Sprang off the Shovel of Death 30 Times in 30 Years." That article was followed by an interview on a major German television show.

Within the United States, I was invited to be a featured guest on another big daytime program, *The Maury Show*, in New York City. Maury Povich seemed like a fairly nice guy. When he introduced me on his show, he stated, "Bill Goss has gone through every disaster imaginable, and he's lived to talk about it." After he interviewed me, he laughingly concluded with, "I don't believe this!," which, of course, made me laugh, because to me, since I lived it, there's nothing unbelievable about it at all.

After that show, I received some very nice letters from people around the country who found my story both educational and inspirational. I started to learn that on the radio, almost every listener has been touched in some way by cancer. The same with television: every viewer is either battling or will be battling or is afraid of battling cancer. Or they have lost at least one person close to them to this very tricky and complex disease. Some people I have met have counted on their fingers for me the number of people in their families who had died from cancer. When they got to their tenth finger, almost embarrassed, they stopped counting.

Many of my personal stories, the individual close brushes with death and catastrophes that I had recounted in *The Luckiest Unlucky Man Alive*, were re-created by actors on Japan's top-rated television show, *Unbelievable*, on the Fuji Network.

One of the surprising things about this extensive re-creation of my life on Japanese television was that they depicted so many of my near brushes with death, except one. The one I personally consider the most important one. They never mentioned my near-fatal collision with cancer. One of my Japanese friends said that in certain Asian cultures, the word cancer is still spoken in a hushed way, like it was in the United States thirty years ago, when people would have whispered behind your back, "That guy over there has the big C," feeling unable to say *cancer* out loud in polite society.

But Rocky wasn't a part of this feature show in Japan either. I tried to tell the Rockster one night at dinner, that his not being on the show was nothing he should take personally. That the Japanese didn't know what flying squirrels were because there weren't any in Japan. That's when Brian piped in with, "Did they eat them all, Dad?"

But finally Rocky got lucky. Finally he got his own chance for a taste of the big time. Finally the Rock got the call. He was invited to be a guest on *Sally Jessy Raphael*, with this particular show being totally dedicated to one surprisingly nice topic—animals and the people who love them. The title of this episode was "Sally's Most Amazing Pets."

Sally, a big animal lover, had already read a little bit about Rocky in *The Luckiest Unlucky Man Alive*. She now wanted us to be guests on her show in New York City, also known as the Big Apple. But this time, I felt I was just coming along for the ride, maybe as an interpreter.

This time, Rocky was going to be the star of the show, not me.

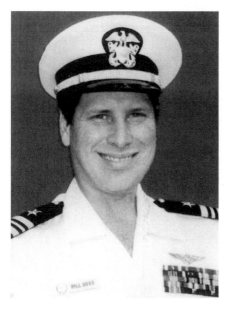

*T*he author right before cancer surgery, 1994.

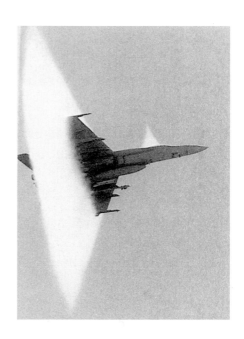

*T*his is what an F-18 Hornet looks like when it breaks the sound barrier. Notice the moisture condensing around the aircraft.

*I*mmediately after going supersonic in the F-18 Hornet with friend Bruce Hilgartner, a former U.S. Marine Corps fighter pilot.

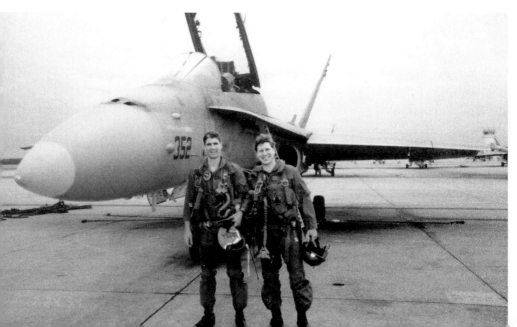

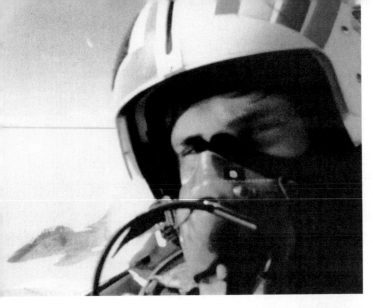

*F*lying the TA-4 Skyhawk jet in formation over Texas.

*T*he author on the navigation bridge of the nuclear aircraft carrier USS *Carl Vinson*, where he served as the assistant navigator and as underway officer of the deck.

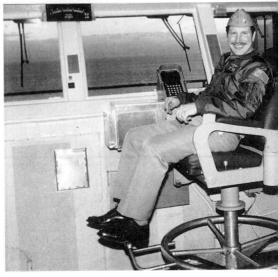

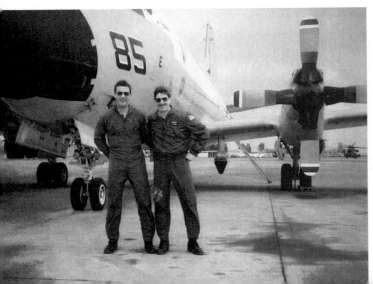

*W*ith former Navy pilot Jay Hanson in front of a Navy P-3 Orion spy plane they both piloted.

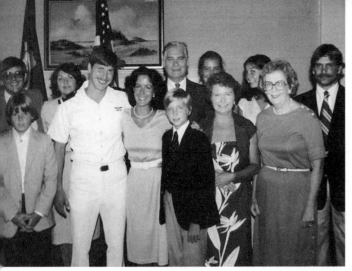

*T*he author celebrating with family and friends in the officer's club at the naval air station in Corpus Christi, Texas, right after receiving his coveted Navy Pilot Wings of Gold.

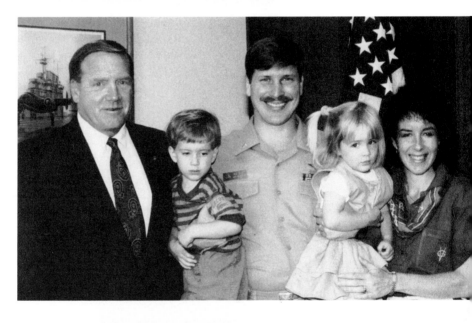

*J*ust after getting promoted to Lieutenant Commander, with cousin Tom Clark, Brian, Christie, and Peggy.

*C*hristie—all smiles with her dad after surgery.

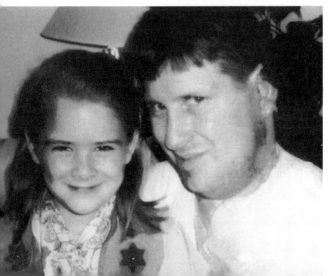

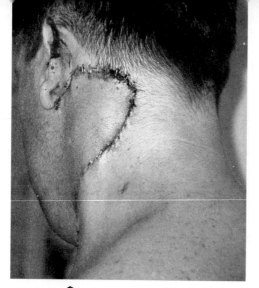

*O*n the road to recovery a few weeks after surgery.

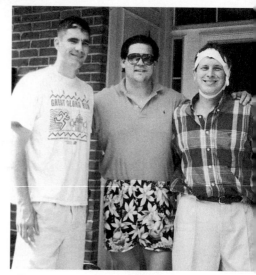

*F*ormer U.S. Marine Corps pilot Bruce Hilgartner and Jeff Marcketta with the author, a day after he had reconstructive surgery on his left ear.

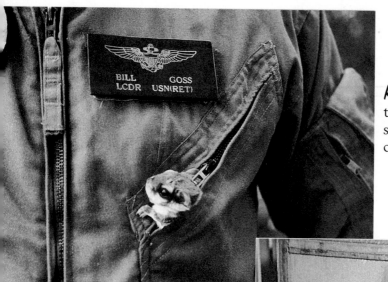

*R*ocky peering out of the author's flight suit. What a great copilot!

*R*ocky waking up and keeping an eye on his prized possession—a big red apple.

*C*hristie's "coonskin cap" is really Rocky hiding in her hair.

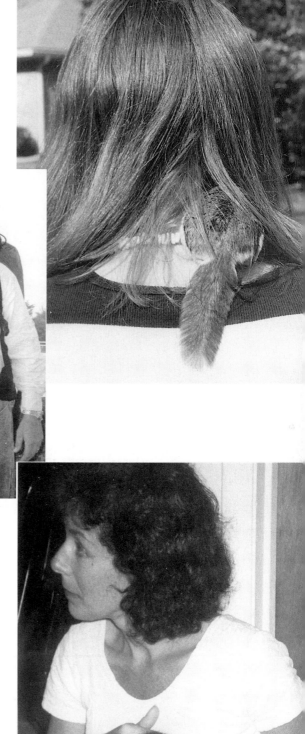

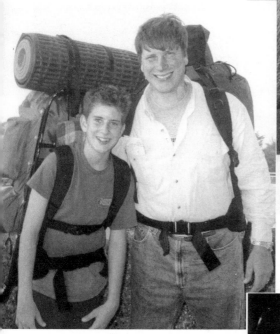

*B*rian hiking with his dad on the highest part of the Appalachian Trail.

*P*eggy with one of the raccoon babies she and Bill helped nurse back to health.

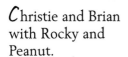

*C*hristie and Brian with Rocky and Peanut.

*R*ocky keeping an eye on things.

*B*rian and Christie face-to-face with a teenage manatee just about their age in manatee years.

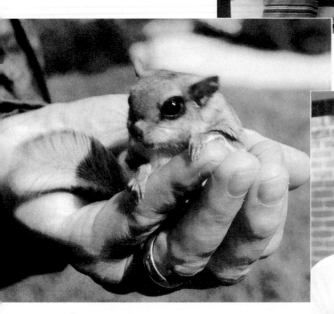

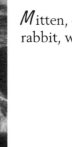

*M*itten, our ten-year-old rabbit, with Christie.

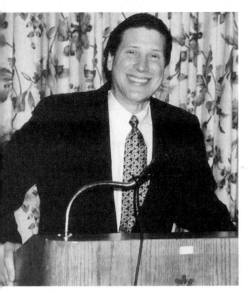

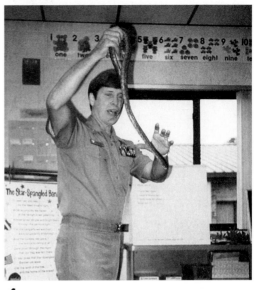

*T*he author giving a speech to the American Cancer Society.

*A*t a Florida school giving a lecture on snakes—and holding a five-foot red rat snake.

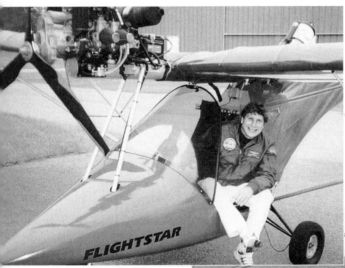

*T*he author and Rocky in the ultra-lite plane they flew for the Discovery Channel's Animal Planet.

*W*ith Peggy, being interviewed for the Discovery Channel.

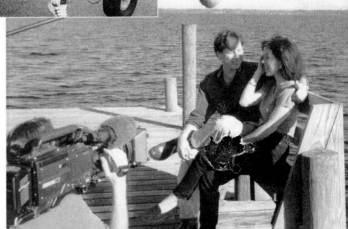

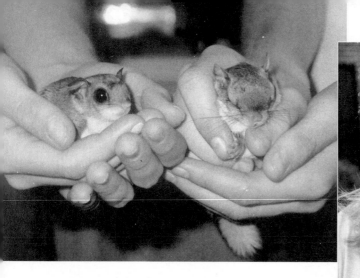

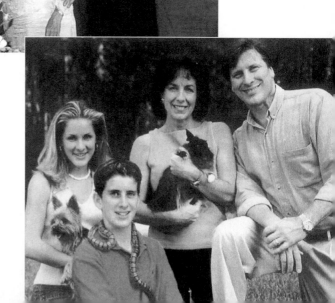

*R*ocky and Bitsy meet for the first time. She's shy! Her eyes are closed.

*C*hristie with Bitsy.

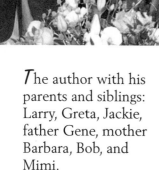

*T*he author with his parents and siblings: Larry, Greta, Jackie, father Gene, mother Barbara, Bob, and Mimi.

*P*ortrait of a happy family. *(Photo by Brian Velenchenko)*

10

Rocky Flies to the Big Apple . . . in First-Class Style

When the producer of *Sally Jessy Raphael* called to help book a flight for Rocky and me to fly up to New York City, a dilemma immediately began. You might think major daytime television shows fly their guests first class when they are invited to be on a show, but that's not true, unless the person is a big movie star, and there are a lot fewer of them than you might think. Television producers operate under very strict budget constraints, and they will do anything they can to demonstrate to their executive producers that they are actually trying to save money.

So, before the producer turned me over to the show's travel coordinator, I told her the truth—that I would need a first-class ticket from Jacksonville to New York City if they wanted me to bring Rocky.

"Why?" she exclaimed.

"Well, where is Rocky going to sit?" I asked.

"Um . . . Good question . . . how big is this animal?"

"Seriously, I checked the airline regulations and it appears that only dogs, cats, birds, and pigs can fly on commercial jets in the United States," I replied.

"Uh-oh," she groaned. "They really want Rocky for this show."

"No cause for worry," I said. "I've got a plan. If you fly Rocky and me first class, I will be almost guaranteed to have an empty overhead bin since first class always boards first. However, if you book us coach, the likelihood of being able to put Rocky in the overhead compartment directly above me is much more remote.

"But, even more important, stress and anxiety caused by loud noises, sudden movements, dramatic temperature changes (maybe even fear of flying) have been known to cause flying squirrels to have heart attacks and die of fright right there on the spot. That's the last thing in the world I would want to happen to my little Rocky. And if I pulled a small dead squirrel out of my pocket in front of all those people, it would not only break my heart, but I think Sally might get a little upset too—maybe even at you."

"I think I'm getting your drift, Lieutenant Commander Goss. Let me talk with our executive producer and I'll get right back to you."

An hour later, I got a call from a more senior producer. "Commander, how many flying squirrels have flown first class to the Big Apple?"

"I'm not sure, but let me guess—none?"

"Well," she laughed, somewhat triumphantly, "that's what we figured, too. Looks like Rocky's gonna be the first."

A few days later, Rocky was in my left shirt pocket, his head poking out the top, carefully observing the cars speeding by on I-95, as we drove my beautiful old gray Porsche to Jacksonville International Airport.

When I arrived, I immediately went into the men's room and slipped Rocky out of my pocket and into a small portable cage, which I then placed into a black carry-on bag. Going through security was a breeze. You'd think that a wire cage in a carry-on bag with a live flying squirrel would have triggered some kind of alert, wouldn't you? But nothing.

Once in the first-class cabin, I gently placed this bag in the bin directly above me, as we prepared for the two-hour flight to New York. I'm sure I heard Rocky chirp a few times overhead as the flight attendant offered me some roasted nuts, though she obviously didn't have a clue. I mean, really, how many times had she heard a flying squirrel chirp on her plane?

Maybe the chirping was Rocky's way of saying to the flight attendant, "Hey you—up here! What about me, lady? I'm a squirrel—I love roasted nuts."

If Rocky got a kick out of the flight, he got an even bigger kick out of the black-stretch limousine driver holding a sign above his head by the luggage pickup. The cardboard sign read simply, MR. ROCKY. Boy, do those producers know how to rub it in.

The poor limousine driver. As he drove us to the studio near Radio City Music Hall, in the busy New York City traffic, he kept looking in the rearview mirror, wondering if his eyes were playing tricks on him, as he saw this furry little thing pop out of my shirt pocket, shoot up to the top of my head, and then shoot back down again into my pocket. But what can I say—Rocky was pumped. It was the Rock's first road trip and likely his first and last visit to the Big Apple.

The night before, Peggy had slipped a big red apple into Rocky's cage. Rocky immediately leaped over to it, wrapped his arms around it, and, using his tiny paws, started to nibble excitedly. His eyes were a lot bigger than his stomach. "Rocky, the next big apple you see is going to be a whole lot bigger than that one," Peggy said, laughing.

The giant stretch limo, designed specifically for Rocky and me, seemed like overkill for only the two of us. But after our royal treatment on Continental Airlines, with our noses held high, we started enjoying the good life. Not bad for a former garbage man who used to park cars on weekends at Yankee Stadium, I figured. But I knew, in my heart of hearts, that without this tiny rodent by my side, I was nothing, at least to these people.

When we arrived in front of our hotel, next door to the studio where the show was to be taped, I was surprised to see another black stretch limousine, just like the one Rocky and I were in. Both rear doors were wide open, with a large man obviously trying very hard to push something out of the limo with all his might, and another man on the other side of the limo trying to pull something out of the other rear door, also with all his might.

Hmmm, I thought to myself. This might be interesting.

Suddenly, with a large yell, the pulling man fell backward, and this huge pig popped out of the back of the limousine and almost landed on top of the guy. "Holy smokes, Rocky, will you look at that!" I exclaimed to the Rockster, as he watched this human–pig spectacle with me in utter amazement. It turned out this big potbellied pig was going to be a guest on *Sally* as well. This really was going to be a show about all creatures, great *and* small.

Checking in to the beautiful hotel, the woman behind the

registration counter handed me a key for the room that the show had reserved for Rocky and me.

I smiled at her and said jokingly, "I promise we won't act like pigs."

Quickly she responded, "You and Rocky are getting our five-star treatment. We've had plenty of pigs stay here—and even some rock stars—but never a flying squirrel."

Riding the elevator up to the very top of the hotel, I unlocked the door to our hotel room. Wow—it was like a presidential suite! Absolutely gorgeous! There was a huge living room, decorated with gorgeous antiques, and Rocky and I had our own attaching bedrooms. Both had balconies with an open and direct view of the entire Empire State Building, just a few blocks away.

Until the twin towers of the World Trade Center were built in the early 1970s, it was the tallest building in the world. Tonight it was brightly illuminated in its traditional holiday red and green Christmas lights from its first floor, on Fifth Avenue and Thirty-fourth Street, to its pointed spire over one hundred stories up. What a spectacular skyline—talk about a room with a view!

Two bedrooms—Rocky's late-night chirping wouldn't be keeping me up after all. I called Peggy right away to tell her that Rocky and I had arrived safely. Wisely, I downplayed the hotel room's elegance—I didn't want to make Peggy feel bad. I had asked her to come with me, but she had decided it would be best if she stayed home with Brian and Christie. This was far too romantic a suite to be wasted on two guys like Rocky and me. Peggy would have loved it, and I felt bad that she, and maybe even the kids, weren't here to enjoy it with us.

While talking with her on the phone, I let Rocky run around the master bedroom to blow off some steam after his long flight up the eastern seaboard. Suddenly, he shot out through the crack of the master-bedroom door. "Peggy, I've got to go!" I screamed as I hung up, trying to get Rocky before he blasted out the open balcony door to his probable death hundreds of feet below. Luckily, I snagged him just as he was about to hit the balcony and enter flying squirrel eternity with all the other little angels. Even if he had safely glided all the way down to the street, he was sure to be flattened by a speeding yellow taxi.

If Rocky ever had high anxiety, this is the day it should have manifested itself. Since it was winter and already nighttime in the city, my nocturnal friend was coming to life, like Wolfman or Dr. Jekyll and Mr. Hyde, a hypermanic little monster in every sense of the word. His black eyes bulging hugely, like a hamster with an overactive thyroid, Rocky was really excited about this trip—maybe too excited.

If this was how he was now, how would the Rock be twelve hours later, sitting next to a big fat pig, on his first TV show, being interviewed by Sally Jessy Raphael (who, by the way, with her big red-framed spectacles, looked a whole lot like Rocky)?

Would Rocky be dead asleep during tomorrow's show—or even worse, would Rocky be *dead*? Or would he be insanely uncontrollable like he was right now?

Ever since witnessing the incident with the hog, I was starting to get a little nervous about things. Maybe I had accepted this invitation just a little too hastily. One thing was certain. If I returned home with a dead squirrel, Peggy was going to kill me.

Despite Rocky's plans for a wild night, after talking with Peggy again, this time a little more calmly, I decided to call it an early evening, with that gorgeous view of the brightly lit Empire State Building right out my balcony window.

The following morning, after breakfast in bed (thanks, Sally!), with Rocky stealing all the strawberries, of course—I took a shower and got Rocky ready to rock and roll. The Rockster had been up all night, wilder than ever, shooting and bouncing like a pinball over the four walls of his cage. And now—after eating the choice pieces from my fruit plate—he was comatose, in hypoglycemic shock, curled up into a plum-sized furball, sleeping on a bed of cotton, on the bottom of a little brown gift box from Macy's.

"Great, just great, Rocky . . . you're all partied out. Nice job, buddy," I said facetiously, now loath to walk across the street to the studio, to be there at the appointed time, to meet my man-ifest destiny with a pig.

Rocky's gonna be worthless and the producer's gonna mur-der me, I thought as I was led up to the Green Room to get prepared for the show.

The makeup artist looked at me in the mirror and then peered at Rocky in the little Macy's gift box.

"You look okay, but your squirrel's got bags under his eyes," she joked, as she sprayed some foo-foo juice on my hair to keep it from falling into my eyes during the show.

"Your rodent looks kind of greasy; aren't they supposed to preen themselves?" she added.

"Normally, yes, but he had a big night," I replied halfheart-edly. "Is there anything you can do for him?"

"Well, a few minutes ago I put some smelling salts under the nose of a pig, but unfortunately he ate them all."

"Thanks. I think Rocky will get by. When will he be going on?" I asked.

"Right now—straight down that hall to the right. And, next time, Mr. Goss, you might want to be a little more responsible with your squirrel, if you know what I mean."

"Five, four, three, two, one . . ."

Sally Jessy Raphael suddenly emerged from the side door of the large room that contained the studio audience. Behind her she was pulling a little red wagon packed full of adorable puppies. This woman's good, I thought to myself, as she handed puppies to the audience to hold during the taping.

Reading from the TelePrompTer, she began her opening introduction: "If you've ever had a pet, you probably know that special bond that develops between an animal and its owner. Well, today you're going to meet some animals that have done some truly amazing things. You're going to meet a pig named Honeymoon that saved its owner's life and a dog named Ginny that has made a career out of saving over four hundred cats' lives.

"My first guest is a veterinarian and author of *Chicken Soup for the Pet Lover's Soul,* so please welcome Dr. Marty Becker. We're also going to get started with a guest whose story appears in the book. His name is Bill Goss, and he has a flying squirrel named Rocky."

With that, Sally and I began a dialogue in front of her live audience. She peppered me with questions like, "Bill, what's a flying squirrel? I heard you had a life-threatening illness and Rocky helped you out—is that true? I hear Rocky's like a member of your family—I'd love to meet him—can you take him out?"

I answered her questions and then opened Rocky's cage door, not knowing whether the Rockster would really come to life or not, after his wild behavior last night.

Above his open cage door, I crumbled a cellophane bag full of pecans, a sound that is normally like music to his ears. Would he still respond to it?

Absolutely! As soon as Rocky heard the sound, he jumped

out of the cage, then leaped onto my sport coat and on up my chest to my left shoulder. From there he gingerly crawled over to my face to say hello, and then, in front of a live studio audience on an internationally broadcast television show, he gave me a tender little kiss on the lips.

It was so adorable that Sally and her audience just melted. He then sat on my shoulder as Sally, now totally entranced by Rocky's magnetic powers, continued to ask me questions while staring adoringly at Rocky. I explained how, after my extensive cancer surgery, Rocky would sleep on my scars underneath my bathrobe as I read the morning paper, and how I thought that helped me recover so much better and so much faster than normal.

Furthermore, it seemed to help my deep surgical scars just melt away. Just as I finished making that last statement, Rocky, as if on cue, took a look at Sally, then climbed up to my neck and dove under my shirt. Sally and the audience watched this little lump under my shirt move around until it had settled at the base of my neck, the site of my few remaining scars. Again, Sally and the audience dissolved at the utter cuteness of it all. Even I was stunned. How could such a tiny creature perform in front of millions of viewers on cue, almost as if reading their minds, like a classically trained stage actor. Delighted by the remarkable magic of the moment, Sally instantly exclaimed, "There it is—on live TV!"

She then talked with the man sitting next to me, America's best-loved veterinarian and now a great friend of mine, Dr. Marty Becker. Marty explained how powerful the bond is between people and their pets, especially in regard to Rocky and me and the other guests who followed, like Phillip Gonzales and Ginny, the famous dog that saves cats, and Honeymoon, the pig that squealed, oinked, and kicked around so much that her owners woke up just in the nick of time to save themselves from a raging house fire.

The grand finale of the show was my friend Dr. Marty Becker handing over a giant-sized check to the American Society for the Prevention of Cruelty to Animals (ASPCA) for the amount of $125,000. This was a donation from himself, his three coauthors, and the publisher of *Chicken Soup for the Pet Lover's Soul*.

This was widely regarded by many as one of the nicest and most endearing shows that Sally Jessy Raphael ever did.

After the show, everyone said their goodbyes and we were all told what time to be downstairs to meet our limousines for the trip back to Newark airport. I had arranged for a later flight so I could spend the day with my parents out at the old Goss homestead.

At the suggestion of Anne Sellaro, Dr. Becker's talented publicist, Sally's producers told me that instead of the quick drive to the airport, the limousine could drive Rocky and me to my parents' home in the township of Millburn-Short Hills, New Jersey. So, after watching the entertaining spectacle of Honeymoon the Pig getting rammed back into a limousine for her trip home, Rocky and I were on our way.

An hour after leaving New York City, we drove up to the top of Cypress Street and then pulled into the driveway of a gray with white trim, cedar-shingled three-story house, my old boyhood home. The yard still heavily wooded with large trees, I reflected for a moment on the late-night shadows flitting among the big oak trees like tiny ghostlike Frisbees across our front and back lawn. My grade-school buddies Rat, Cubie, Boobus, Foof, Gureenie, Duvalle, and I recognized the bats, owls, and whippoorwills zooming through the evening sky. But these other things, we were just spooked and mystified by them—we generally just thought we were seeing things.

Then I looked up the hill at the 4,000-acre forest where I had spent so much of my boyhood hiking with my parents, siblings, friends, and cousins. My eyes and ears were trained to be ever alert to the slightest movement or rustling in the leaves. It could be anything—perhaps just the wind, but quite possibly an animal that I might be able to observe for a moment. Or, if I was really lucky, one that I could catch and take home in my pocket for a spell, if I could sneak it past my parents on the way up the stairs to my bedroom. My parents had been tolerant of so many aspects of my being, especially when it came to my roomful of live animals on the second floor of our house, that it served as a reminder to me that maybe I should be likewise with my own children.

And now, more than ever, my parents' front yard was being invaded daily by a host of interesting and friendly animals, from occasional large herds of white-tailed deer to foraging woodchucks, rabbits, skunks, possums, fox, and even wild turkeys. And this is all happening in a relatively urban environment. It's a stunning example of humans and animals living together in a unique and vibrant new kind of way, an urban wildlife kind of way that is becoming more and more common. In fact, in many ways, we are starting to see an explosion of wildlife throughout America, in our towns and sometimes even our cities.

A movement in a window of my parents' home brought me back to present times and I saw my mother cup her hands in front of her eyes to get a better look out their upstairs bedroom window. A moment later, the front door opened and out she came to greet me as I climbed out of the back of the limo with Rocky in a small handheld cage.

In just a matter of seconds—I knew it wouldn't take long—Mom's curiosity got the better of her, and she stuck her head inside the back of the stretch limo, expecting to see somebody important inside. Half joking—and half disappointed—to find the limo empty, Mom pulled her head out to look me directly in the eyes and then asked, "Come on now, Billy—all this for a squirrel?"

11

Rocky's Roommates and Other Strange Bedfellows

*A*fter the Sally show, things slowed down for the holidays. Peggy, Brian, Christie, and I were rather amused when we discovered how much Rocky enjoyed climbing around in our Christmas tree. That is, until he made it up to the top and saw the golden angel ornament plunked on her traditional spot at the tree's peak. Rocky met her eye to eye and then gave us a look like he was thinking, Heh, what's *she* doing up here? I'm the little angel in this house!

During this winter season I went in for a second CAT scan. For malignant melanoma survivors with a history of deep tumors, an annual or biannual CAT scan is one of the recommended follow-up procedures. After a few days to get the digital images read by the radiology department and then transcribed into a written report, I received a copy of it. Thankfully, I was still cancer-free.

A full-page story was written by Ron Word, a senior writer for the Associated Press, about some of the lucky and unlucky challenges I'd been through over the past thirty years. It was a well-written article and it quickly got picked up by many of the major and local newspapers across the country. The *Chicago Tribune*, the *Los Angeles Times*, *The Washington Post*, the *Orlando Sentinel*, the *Detroit News*, the *Seattle Times*, the *St. Petersburg Times*, the *Las Vegas Review* and the *San Francisco Examiner* were some of the larger papers to run the story. Some independent writers from the *New Jersey Star-Ledger*, the *Chattanooga Times*, the *Florida Times-Union* and the infamous *Bikini* magazine also wrote articles focusing on my struggle and victory against cancer.

As well-written as these articles were, when my life was laid out by the writers, even in extensive detail, they almost failed to include the one thing that has always been a central part of my life since I was a small boy—animals. Especially wild animals.

In many ways, if I had to pick one specific thing I thoroughly enjoy—other than the obvious stuff men and women enjoy—it would be that I love to observe wild animals in their native habitats, the rarer and more difficult to observe the better. So many of my most interesting experiences have been while in pursuit of wild things, not to kill but simply to observe them, always with the possibility to learn something new.

I wanted to be tracking and observing wild animals all the time and that is not an easy thing to do when you're not born independently wealthy. So, when the opportunity availed itself, I brought animals into our home just so I could continue my favorite hobby—the study of animal behavior—even right after getting home from a long mission flying as a Navy pilot. I have always found watching animals extremely relaxing and yet, at the same time, intensely interesting.

When Peggy and I first met, she was not particularly interested in wild animals, but she had a tremendous love for domestic animals, especially dogs. When she was little girl growing up with her six siblings in South Orange, New Jersey, Peggy's family had a dog named Bingo. Peggy lived and breathed for Bingo, and so did her older brother, Tony, and her younger brother, Chris. They used to dress up Bingo, a medium-sized, black-and-white Heinz 57 mutt with a great disposition, and treat him like he was royalty. In fact, they treated him more like a king, the head of royalty, with little parades for him around the house, and they even made a throne and a crown for him.

Peggy was a real dog lover then and still is today. But she's always preferred to have only one dog and shower it with attention, rather than have a couple of dogs and worry about spreading the special one-on-one relationship too thin.

I, on the other hand, liked to have a whole lot of animals around, to observe the diversity of all the different species. Always more of a linear thinker than Peggy (she was much more into having a warm and loving relationship with a pet), I was interested in watching a lot of wild animals do their thing. That's why my relationship with Rocky is so different than with most other animals—we have a really deep and special relationship—an actual love for each other.

Peggy and I have had a lot of fun and fascinating animals come through our home over the past twenty years. Some have been roommates of Rocky's. Some came and went long before Rocky first fell from the sky and into our lives. Here are a few of those animals' stories.

The first animals that came into Peggy's and my life together was in Corpus Christi, Texas, right after I'd completed Aviation Officer Candidate School (AOCS), the same program that was portrayed in the Academy Award–winning movie *An Officer and a Gentleman.*

Peggy, who had graduated college a few months earlier like myself, had flown down from New Jersey to see me get commissioned as an ensign in the United States Navy. Shortly after the traditional commissioning ceremony on the parade grounds, Peggy and I, rather jubilant after I had survived the academically and physically demanding sixteen-week program run by U.S. Marine Corps drill instructors, we got married. We were just plain head over heels in love and didn't feel like not being married to each other for one more second.

Right after that, for the first time together as a married couple, we jumped into my old Volvo and drove nine hundred miles to Corpus Christi, Texas, where I was to begin my training as a Navy pilot.

Rather quickly, we had a problem. A snake problem. You see, my roommates at Rutgers had been taking care of the four large snakes I had in the fraternity-like house I shared with three other students and one professor.

These snakes had come in handy on more than one occasion. I actually did two research papers at Rutgers using these snakes. One of the papers was on how to trigger the breeding of endangered northern pine snakes by providing them with a simulated rather than a true period of hibernation. I accomplished the simulated hibernation by putting them, for several weeks at a time, in my roommates' and my refrigerator. They hissed like crazy anytime anyone opened or closed the refrigerator, with most people thinking we had a freon gas leak. I got an A on that paper—my ecology professor thought it was a rather novel idea.

Peggy, to me a true sign of love, agreed to keep my pet

snakes in her apartment while I was completing AOCS training in Pensacola. Since our elopement was completely unplanned, the result of unbridled passion, youthful impulsiveness, and being wildly in love, we were now driving to Texas, but my pet snakes were still in New Jersey in Peg's apartment.

When we finally got to Texas and moved into the Navy Base housing, Peggy flew back to New Jersey to pick up all her stuff, try to explain our elopement to her parents and mine, and then return—with a lot of luggage and four snakes in tow. What a trooper she was. I thought facing Navy flight instructors was hard—facing her parents and then my parents had to be ten times harder.

So, while learning to fly Navy airplanes, I had my pet snakes at home to help me relax after a tough day of flying the grossly overpowered 1,425-horsepower single-engine T-28 Trojan.

Peggy also had brought back a pet box turtle we had named Hercules. Peggy wasn't such a big fan of the snakes, but she loved Hercules, who would crawl across the kitchen floor when we sat down at the kitchen table to eat. He would then rear his neck and head up so high, trying to get our attention to feed him, begging just like a dog. If that didn't work, he'd start jumping, sometimes so high and brazenly he'd end up flipping over onto his back. He was hilarious.

Hercules ended up with another shelled friend, a few months later, who was about ten times his size. It was a Texas desert tortoise who started showing up in our backyard at dusk, eating our grass, and later on, the bread and table scraps we put out for him. Both he and Hercules often had free rein of our house, unlike the snakes, who were such extraordinary escape artists that they were always in their cages unless I was holding them.

Eventually, after receiving my coveted Navy Pilot Wings of Gold, I got my orders to fly P-3 Orion aircraft home based out of the naval air station in Brunswick, Maine. The desert tortoise was returned to the wilds of our backyard to cheer up the next Navy pilot and spouse who moved in after us. And Hercules the box turtle was returned to a heavily wooded area of New Jersey near where I had originally found him attempting to cross a busy road.

I had promised my wife the dog lover that we would get a puppy as soon as we moved into a place where we were going to stay put for an extended period of time. We had both agreed it wouldn't be good for us to get a puppy while we were still on the move, without a place to truly call home, especially with our potential to be transferred overseas. So we hadn't yet acquired the promised puppy. But I could see how it was wearing on Peggy, not having a cute little dog running to the door to greet her when she came in. Or not having a dog's head on her lap as she read or watched television at night. When I was not flying, I had to be studying almost constantly, memorizing vast quantities of new flight procedures, new aircraft mechanical systems, course rules, weapon systems, standard operating procedures—there was always something I needed to learn yesterday so I'd be prepared for today's test. And, without a doubt, sometimes all my intense studying made our house a lonely place for Peggy, even when I was home. Peggy needed a dog and needed one quick.

After six months of advanced flight training in Jacksonville, Florida, Peggy and I drove our old Volvo to Maine. We watched the odometer click past 200,000 miles as we pulled into the driveway of the one-hundred-year-old three-story house we had just purchased. Located in Bath, Maine, our home was just a few blocks from the Bath Iron Works, an active shipyard famous for the Navy destroyers and cruisers it made in record-setting time during WW II.

Still on vacation, I checked in with my new squadron, Patrol Squadron Eight, a few miles down the road at the naval air station in the town of Brunswick. I got back to Bath to help Peggy unpack and set up our new house.

When I walked through the front door, she had the look. I knew that look, a look that I was never going to get out of my head until I had righted some wrong I had done. But first I needed to know what that was. What had I said or done to have fallen from that pedestal all loving spouses like to imagine themselves seated high upon at least once in a while?

"Bill, you promised."

"I promised what, Peggy?"

"You promised me we'd get a dog as soon as we settled in to a place for a while. This is that place, honey," she said, looking both radiant and imploring at the same time.

"Peg, the car's not even unpacked yet."

"Well, we'll just have to get a smaller dog then. Let's go—there's a pet store about ten minutes from here."

An hour later, we were back home with a tiny black-haired Yorkshire terrier puppy, and about four hundred dollars poorer. Looking at Peggy, who was looking adoringly at her—I mean our—new puppy sound asleep inside one of my sneakers, I did some quick math. About fifty dollars an ounce, I figured.

Pilots are reputed to be notoriously cheap.

The puppy was so tiny and lackluster that I had mentioned to the pet store sales clerk that the dog appeared sick.

"Oh, you don't think this one has personality, do you? Well, just watch this," she said, scooping up another puppy and putting it with the tiny Yorkie. Instantly, the Yorkie came to life, gleefully playing, smiling with its eyes, and with her snow-white puppy teeth.

"Too cute. There's no way out for me this time. I might as well take out my checkbook right now," I thought to myself.

"What do you think, Bill?" Peggy asked, but I didn't really hear any question in her voice.

"That's the one, honey. I like the way she kind of scoots around. Happy early birthday—way early."

Scooter grew into five pounds of love, high energy, and entertainment, and we became the very best of friends. I adored her. Over the next four years, because I was so far from home on extended six-month deployments and detachments to Bermuda, Iceland, the Azores, Sicily, Brazil, and Spain, Scooter became an absolutely critical factor in the early survival years of our marriage.

If it hadn't been for Scooter, the loneliness of that big old house might have proved too much for Peggy, as it had for so many other spouses of Navy men and women.

When I was far away, flying (spying) on Soviet submarines from distant locations around the world, I always had the camaraderie of my crew and of my fellow naval officers. Peggy had little of that. Besides an occasional get-together with other Navy wives, she spent a lot of time alone. But Scooter was always there by her side, twenty-four hours a day, seven days a week, as both her best friend and as a great little watch-dog.

Scooter used to do a lot of funny things. For three years, she would pull all the mail through the slot in our front door just at the moment the mailman was inserting it through, terrorizing the poor postal worker and always damaging our mail. The wonderful retired man next door to us, Len

Thombs, who adored Scooter, used to sit by his living room window whenever he could, just waiting to see the mailman put the mail through our slot and then walk away muttering to himself.

One day, when I heard the familiar *clink-clink* of our brass mail slot being pushed open, I quietly snuck up to the front door and watched as Scooter growled ferociously as she tore the envelopes right out of the mailman's fingers.

When no more mail was forthcoming through the slot, I let tiny growling Scooter out the front door to chase after the mailman, who suddenly turned to look at Scooter, then at me, first with a start, then with a bemused look on his face, like he'd just been had.

"Do you mean to tell me that this is the dog making all of those ferocious sounds on the other side of the door? Why, why, that's nothing but a rat—a rat dog!" the mailman said. "And please, tell me, what the hell does your mail look like after your rat dog gets through with it?"

"Through rain and sleet and snow . . . and rat dogs . . ." I said to the mailman. "Besides, Scooter only eats the bills—she cashes the checks."

At the age of four, Scooter transferred with Peggy and me back to Texas when I became an instructor, teaching student Navy pilots how to fly multiengine airplanes under engine-out conditions (flying the Navy T-44 Pegasus airplane) and how to use advanced navigation systems.

When Christie and Brian were born, Scooter became like their little guardian angel. And they adored her as well. Brian and Christie loved to watch her fish with me in the canal behind our home on Padre Island, Texas. When Scooter would see my line tighten up, she would peer into the salt water and stare at the spot where the fishing line was coming out. At the moment she saw that a fish was really attached to my line, Scooter would dive five to ten feet off the wall we were fishing from to catch the fish in her teeth. This was one amazing little dog.

Yorkies were first bred in Great Britain hundreds of years ago specifically to kill rats—to be ratters. But Peggy and I are convinced that something went awry in Scooter's case, because she appeared to have been bred to kill fish, not rats. To be a fisher, not a ratter. When some of my macho buddies would see Scooter for the first time, scooting around under everyone's feet, they would laugh and say to me, "Oh, you've got a little rat dog." But then, if we went fishing off the backyard and they saw Scooter dive off our dock or the canal wall to retrieve a fish they'd hooked, they laugh again and say, "She's not a rat dog, she's a fish dog."

Scooter provided us with a lot of laughs and an even greater amount of love over the thirteen years she was with our family. Once, while she was surveying the salt water canal for surfacing redfish, she started barking insanely. Something was obviously down in the water, but was not in our visual line of sight. Peggy and I ran down to the water's edge to see what was in there.

The poor thing! It was a little half-grown ground squirrel that was treading water, and probably had been for a long time, unable to get itself out of the canal due to the steep concrete walls.

"Scooter, you saved a squirrel!" we praised her with, as we fished out the thoroughly bedraggled and near-dead ground squirrel. "'Good squirrel dog," I said to her, raising her from the ranks of rat dog and fish dog. Not knowing quite how to administer squirrel CPR, I pushed the tip of my index finger on the catatonic little creature's stomach.

Salt water squirted out from the poor guy's mouth. I did that a couple of more times, then we put Mr. Squirrel into a box with some food and fresh water, which Peggy had prepared for him.

This squirrel looked dreadful. His eyes were all swollen and sealed shut from the hours he'd been half submerged in the salt water. Peggy and I prayed for the little guy, prayed to St. Squirrelly, the patron saint of all of God's little creatures, seated right up there next to St. Joan of Arc. A few hours later, Mr. Squirrel's eyes were half open and somewhat alert. Lying on his side, looking at me, Mr. Squirrel appeared to have no fear—unusual for a wild ground squirrel, normally extremely alert, ready to bolt at the slightest movement of anything nearby.

"Maybe, just maybe, he's gonna make it," I told Peggy. A few hours later, he was up and about in his temporary new home, eating from Peggy's hand. In a few days, Mr. Squirrel had recovered wonderfully. A week later, after Peggy and I had developed a newfound appreciation for the spirit, toughness, and will to live of a creature small enough to fit in the palm of your hand, we set him free in a wide open field far from the canal.

Amazingly, another creature, much smaller than Mr. Squirrel or even Rocky, was about to fly right into our lives.

Peggy and I had just spent the day at the world-famous San Patricio County Rattlesnake Races, a huge annual event in the Texas tradition of everything being, well, just plain *huge*. Much of the proceeds from the rattlesnake races, the chili cook-off, and the barbecue go to local charities.

The big—let's just say *huge*—and very much alive Texas diamondback rattlesnake I raced fifty yards down the track against other nuts with rattlesnakes, well, my snake lost by just a nose. I took home a second-place ribbon and the knowledge of how to win first place if I ever get back there. Overall, the rattlesnake races had been a wildly fun and unique Texas experience. Peg and I had a lot of laughs about the day's events on the drive back to our home on Padre Island.

After pulling into the garage and stepping out of our old Volvo, Peggy and I both heard a loud buzzing sound. It sounded like a rattlesnake, a noise we'd both become quite familiar with after what we had just been through. Looking around the garage and under the car, finally I noticed this huge june bug banging against the fluorescent light over my work-bench.

Snatching it from the air with my left hand, I suddenly realized it was no june bug. It was a tiny hummingbird.

Weighing in at just a fraction of an ounce, Hummer became a special guest in our house over the next few weeks as we fed him nectar to help him regain his strength for the annual hummingbird migration along the Gulf and then down to Mexico. Some hummingbirds have been known to—instead of flying—hitch a ride by hiding in the back feathers of much larger birds, like geese, that are migrating in the same direction.

In the town of Rockport, Texas, just north of Corpus Christi, there is a big Texas celebration in honor of the millions of southbound hummingbirds passing through.

Rattlesnake races, hummingbird festivals, rodeos, chili cook-offs—Texans just love to throw huge outdoor parties.

Like Mr. Squirrel, whom we found at death's doorstep, Hummer was also very weak, after having beaten himself silly against the light in our garage. But in just a few days, Hummer was again flying in top aviator form.

What a little stick of dynamite he was as he moved around

our house—Hummer could accelerate from zero to thirty mph in the blink of an eye. Moving his wings at over seventy beats per second, he could fly backward, forward, and sideways. He could also remain stationary in flight, hovering like a helicopter as he fed from a sugar-water feeder hung from the ceiling of our guest bedroom.

In the wild, hummingbirds require nectar from as many as five thousand flowers per day, plus a couple of insects, to supply proper nutrition for the incredible metabolism going on within those tiny bodies. Every time a hummingbird dips its long beak into a flower, it also helps to cross-pollinate the plant, a vitally important event in the natural order of our ecosystems.

Hummer was not only cute, he was courageous, defending his bright red hummingbird feeder like a sow bear with cubs. Soon, it was obvious that the little green and red firecracker was ready for release.

Peg and I took him outside into the ever-blowing Corpus Christi wind and I uncupped my hands. He sat there for a moment, quizzically looking at us, like he was saying goodbye. Then he took off. Up he went, straight up over our heads, directly into the noonday sun. We kept watching him as he climbed straight up like the space shuttle. Remarkably, the strongly blowing wind did not deviate his perfectly vertical flight. Finally, thousands of feet above us, Hummer disappeared into the sun—still directly and perfectly overhead, despite the powerfully blowing wind.

How and why Hummer went straight up I'll never understand, but I'd definitely like to, strictly from an aeronautical point of view. A tiny creature weighing less than an ounce flying so precisely straight up into the sky in a heavy wind, only to eventually head south to fly thousands of miles to Mexico, only to return six months later—it's incomprehensible. Even with the most powerful computer microprocessors and the tiniest of batteries, we still can't duplicate, or particularly miniaturize, what is a matter of course for so many of our tiniest marvels of nature, particularly one little hummingbird as he flew south along the Padre Island National Seashore to Mexico.

Living so close to the National Seashore was a naturalist's dream. A favorite event of Peggy's and mine was the seasonal baby sea turtle release. Assisting a National Seashore naturalist, Peggy and I, and sometimes my Aunt Fran from Houston, would follow newly hatched ridley sea turtles, a rare reptilian species, down into the waters of the Gulf of Mexico. Then we'd scoop them up out of the water with a net and return the adorable little hatchlings to the naturalist, who then raised them to a larger size.

It almost seemed mean, but there was a definite method to the madness. Once imprinted by the sights and smells and sounds of their first swim (like Rocky was imprinted by my voice and smell), an extra year's growth in captivity would dramatically help to protect the hatchlings from predators, like seagulls and large fish. They would be released during the following year's hatch as older, stronger, bigger, and possibly even wiser yearlings, helping to ensure the survival of their rapidly diminishing species.

And because of their initial imprinting in local Gulf waters after they had hatched, many of these same turtles would return to Padre Island ten to twenty years later as adults to nest, replenishing the local population of this rare and beautiful creature of the sea.

Peg and I have always felt an obligation to help preserve the God-given natural diversity with which earth has been so fortunately blessed. The way we figure it, once a species is gone, it's gone for good, and it will take the overturning of Heaven and Hell before we see the uniqueness of that creature again. So, we've just got to help out Mother Nature the best we can.

We have so many fond memories of Corpus Christi and Padre Island, particularly because it's where Christie and Brian were conceived and born, allowing Peggy and me to start raising a family of our own, something we'd wanted to do for a few years.

A year after the twins were born, we moved to San Diego for a short aircraft carrier navigation course I had to take, then we headed up to the San Francisco Bay Area so I could start working as the assistant navigator of the nuclear aircraft carrier USS *Carl Vinson*. I had to study and work so hard at this job, unfortunately I had little quality time to spend with my family and no time for animals. With two-year orders, it was just the nature of the job. For a Navy lieutenant, it carried so much responsibility and so many opportunities to screw up, putting countless people's careers and lives on the line, that as professionally fulfilling and as technically fascinating as it was at times, it just was not a lot of fun for Peggy or me.

Again, Scooter saved the day. I was at work or at sea so much of the time. Brian and Christie were being potty trained and had the ability to get into anything and everything. Being twins, they had their own form of twin speak, a unique and acknowledged language that exists between twin babies, but that Peggy and I could not understand. When I was at sea, Peggy swore Brian and Christie were sometimes using their twin speak to plot against her.

Since I wasn't there much, Peggy's only true ally within the confines of the small house we were renting was Scooter. She was combination guard dog and best friend, all packed into five pounds. Incredibly intelligent, she seemed to understand everything Peggy said to her. Like a sheepdog, she completely understood how to herd the twins around the house and up and down the steep stairs that can be really dangerous for toddlers. When I got back from a two-month combat ship exercise in the northern Pacific Ocean, I was shocked to see how Peggy's shoulders and arms had gotten more muscular from picking up and carrying two thirty-pound kids all over the place. She almost looked like Rosie the Riveter from the old WW II posters to buy war bonds. I better not get out of line with her or I'm in for real trouble, I remember thinking to myself.

The only animal we had with us while doing this ship tour in northern California was Scooter. We could barely take care of ourselves, we figured. Who needed the responsibilities of more animals? So one pet was all we had for a spell, even though I was really feeling the need for more. I just felt incomplete—not whole—when I wasn't around a lot of animals.

It was only after we transferred from California to Florida that we finally felt like we could breathe easy again. The cost of living was dramatically lower, and Peggy found a wonderful house to buy that had all the nature and privacy we desired, yet it was still wonderfully set up for the kids to walk to a brand-new elementary school just a few blocks away.

The road just a couple of streets down, Bald Eagle Drive, was aptly named, as there are at least two pairs of nesting bald eagles within a few miles of us. I actually had one pair of bald eagles fly low, slow, and parallel with me for about thirty seconds as I drove down Bald Eagle on the way to work one morning. What a way to start your day! Talk about being pumped—it was awesome!

It was at this house that we started building the Goss

menagerie of old. First of all, the amount of naturally occurring wildlife in Florida is beyond belief for a northern boy. Every year, the cold harsh winters of the Northeast kill off a surprising number of animals due to exposure to the elements, particularly the surprise snowfalls and freezes in late spring. Weather this harsh rarely happens in northern Florida and virtually never happens south of Orlando, so any area in Florida that has bushes or trees is typically teeming with animal life, particular lizards like the green anole and a wide variety of skinks, toads, and tree frogs.

Tiger salamanders are the largest land salamanders in the world at over thirteen inches in length. They are also one of the most beautiful. They not only have the yellow and black pattern of a Bengal tiger, but they stalk and eat nightcrawlers like a big cat. Even though tiger salamanders live throughout North America, they are rarely seen in the wild because they spend most of their time underground. Brian keeps some in a terrarium in his room. They're easy to care for and are one of the more interesting animals to keep as pets, although I'm sure Rocky would argue that.

Amphibians (frogs, toads, and salamanders) are generally not known for their warm and receptive personalities, but as a boy, I always enjoyed catching them in the wild, observing them for a couple of days, then re-releasing them back where I caught them. Frogs and toads generally sit in one spot, waiting for food to come right up to them. When people approach them, frogs and toads usually will either continue sitting right where they are, or they will hop or swim away. And salamanders are typically so small that you can't hold them too much or they will die from being over-handled.

Tigers, on the other hand, are large enough salamanders that you can handle them without worrying about hurting them. A lot like Hercules, our first family box turtle, who learned to beg for food (turtles are reptiles, not amphibians—laying their eggs on land, not in the water) our tigers also quickly came to understand that humans are their meal ticket. So when our salamanders see us or hear us walk into the room, they crawl over to the side of their cage closest to us and start begging for food, until we feed them the large earthworms that we buy from the sporting goods and fishing supplies department at Wal-Mart every week or so. They are becoming much fatter than they ought to be.

Tiger salamanders are one of the most responsive and fascinating cold-blooded animals that you can keep as a pet—and they are relatively easy to care for. Brian's buddies love watching them eat and holding them. They've never seen salamanders quite that big—and probably never will again.

Legless lizards are common in our neighborhood. I usually discover a couple of them mating in our backyard every spring. They look like snakes, but their tails break off easily (they grow back in a few months). The dead giveaway that what is in your yard is a two-foot-long legless lizard and not a snake is that legless lizards have eyelids and ears—snakes have neither. So if you ever see a snake blink— remember—it's not a snake!

It wasn't long after we moved into our new home that Brian, Christie, and I found a couple of beautiful four-foot-long red rat snakes crawling around the neighborhood. Brian ended up putting them together in a large glass aquarium in his room. It turns out Spike and Ike are actually a male and a female. They successfully breed every year. The orange-colored female lays ten to sixteen eggs late each spring. Usually around two-thirds of the eggs successfully hatch out in late summer, with the hatchlings about ten inches long.

Each year, an annual Goss event is for Brian and Christie

and their friends to release the little baby red rat snakes down at the dock to help propagate the species. The red rat snake is particularly valuable to farmers and landowners. One four-foot-long snake is worth thousands of dollars over the course of its life (as long as thirty years) because it will eat hundreds of rats and mice, which have the potential to devour tons of wheat and corn annually.

Speaking of hatchlings, earlier in the book I talked about Little Rascal. Found freshly hatched on their front lawn, with its yolk sac still attached to its bottom shell, our neighbors, Fred and Doty Hussman, brought over a tiny baby box turtle whose bright yellow and orange top shell was no bigger in diameter than a dime. Christie immediately latched on to and named Little Rascal, who, on a steady diet of one earthworm a day, and scraps of food from our kitchen table thrown in for good measure, has grown tenfold.

At least once a day, one of us has to walk by Little Rascal's cage to flip him right side up, after he has flipped himself over while begging for food like a dog, just like Hercules used to do on our kitchen floor in Texas. For a turtle, Little Rascal is quite a character.

And he'd make a very healthy little meal for Tex, our Texas indigo snake, one of the only species of snake that will swallow a small turtle whole, but also likes to do the same with rattlesnakes, cottonmouth water moccasins, and coral snakes. Rocky, as well as Brian's red rat snakes—and even Mitten, our rabbit—would be considered a tasty meal for Tex as well.

Snakes can be notoriously finicky eaters. Because of this, they are often tricky to keep as pets, no matter how fascinating they are to watch as they crawl around their cage. Snakes typically eat only one or two kinds of animals. And, over the course of a year, they probably average only about one decent meal per month because they are such picky eaters. Not the Texas indigo snake. As long as it isn't a plant and isn't a human, and it's some kind of critter small enough for a six-foot-long snake with a big mouth to swallow whole, Tex will consider it lunch. And he likes doing lunch a lot.

Yet, despite his voracious catholic diet and his willingness to try to turn everything into a meal, Tex is as docile and friendly as any pet snake I've ever had. He's absolutely fascinating to observe from an amateur animal behaviorist's point of view. When I let him get some exercise in our backyard, he leisurely crawls along in the grass, his gleaming black and brown scales soaking in the noonday sun. But his tongue starts flicking and his tail starts twitching as he crawls near our pond, suddenly smelling a frog nearby. Tex then arches his neck up like a large cobra, instantly on the hunt, no longer some guy's pet snake but a magnificent and totally focused wild animal, darting his head forward in the grass, attempting to surprise and flush out his amphibious quarry like an undisciplined bird dog.

When sniffing around for frogs by our pond, even Tex has to be careful not to stick his head too deep into the pond water. If he does, the rather hefty largemouth bass that Brian caught a few years ago at a nearby pond, and then transplanted into our pond, might grab Tex by the head and never let go.

Allegedly named after the mounted singing largemouth bass, Big Mouth Billy is even more voracious than Tex. He tries to eat or chase away anything that enters our pond, where he is the self-declared king of the world. I pity the poor wild flying squirrel that misjudges the distance across our pond someday and ends up treading water right in the middle, because Big Mouth Billy is definitely the master of his domain.

For a bass, Big Mouth Billy has unusual tastes—he loves hickory smoked hot dogs and raw hamburgers. He'll sometimes eat them right out of your hand in just a few seconds.

Another place I have to be careful not to let Tex go near is Mitten's cage, home of our long-haired miniature rabbit. With three black paws and one white one, Mitten seemed like the perfect name. A very pretty and sweet rabbit, we got him for Easter when Brian and Christie were in preschool. Mitten, just like Rocky, considers fresh apples and pears a real treat. Sometimes we let him hop around our backyard for exercise, but we always have to worry that a wandering neighborhood dog will come by and be unable to resist its call-of-the-wild tendencies, making short order of our wonderful ten-year-old rabbit.

One other problem when we let Mitten loose in our backyard is that he sometimes discovers an armadillo or gopher tortoise burrow hidden beneath the palmetto fronds. When he does, Mitten usually just can't help himself. He shoots straight down the hole. Typically, we just have to grab a seat and wait for Mitten to pop his head out again, and who knows how long that will take.

Other animals we've taken care of for various periods of time are armadillos (the babies are cute), raccoons (the babies are even cuter than baby armadillos), and even a friend's pet ferret, which was great fun—and absolutely uproarious entertainment. Why? Because when ferrets start to run, their longer hind legs quickly overtake their short front legs, causing them to fall end over end as they build up some speed. They then get up, look at you like it was your fault, then take off again—until they fall end over end once more. Surprisingly, ferrets—which really are like friendly weasels on steroids (and maybe amphetamines)—get along quite well with dogs, especially Yorkshire terriers, because Yorkies and ferrets were bred in Great Britain and elsewhere in Europe to hunt rats together.

Falconry was considered the sport of nobility and kings. Ratting was the sport of everyman. Ferrets and terriers, even today, still compete in ratting tournaments in teamed pairs in those parts of the world where people obviously aren't too fond of rodents (or maybe too fond of them—as food!).

Ferrets are also playfully curious even as adult animals. So are Yorkshire terriers. Scooter maintained the curiosity of a kitten and the playfulness of a puppy throughout her adult life, even until the age of thirteen, when her tiny little heart stopped beating one day.

Her death was rough on all of us, because she had been such a tremendous part of our family. Tearfully, we wrapped her in one of Christie's favorite blankets. Then we all stroked her and talked to her gently. Finally, we placed her in a shoe box and buried her near the waterfall by our pond. We asked Christie and Brian, who were eight years old at the time, what they wanted the world to know about Scooter. Now, above her grave, rests a tombstone that states exactly what they said that day: SCOOTER . . . THE BEST DOG THERE EVER WAS!

In dog years, Scooter had lived to be ninety-one, and we were grateful that she had enjoyed such a long time on earth with us. Scooter's death also reminded us of the temporal nature of life on earth, and how, when our body finally wears out, our essence and spirit have to move on. Scooter also helped us to reflect on how lucky we were that I hadn't died, but instead was incredibly blessed to have survived—and even thrived.

After Scooter passed on, Peggy and I tried to go for a few months without getting another dog, just out of respect for

Scooter, but that proved to be an impossible task for Peggy. She's such a dog person, she feels incomplete if she doesn't have one in her life. (Though I still think a Yorkie is more like a cross between a dog and a cat, rather than 100-percent canine.)

Peggy's argument was that she wanted our next puppy to grow up around a lot of young kids (which Scooter had not done, so consequently she was kind of nervous around other people's children). Peggy also thought, correctly I might add, that it would be good for Christie and Brian to help care for a puppy while they themselves were kind of like puppies. So, when we heard about another litter of Yorkshire terrier puppies that were available for sale, we went to see them. Peggy picked the runt of the litter, a tiny, jet-black female without any energy at all, yet she cost almost twice as much as Scooter had fourteen years earlier, and at half the size. Now, this was a dog who was truly worth her weight in gold. My rationale—at least to my macho Navy pilot buddies who called her Rat Dog Number Two—for such a big expense for such a tiny dog is that they eat so little food compared to a big dog that over the course of their life they're a real bargain.

And when a big dog makes a mess in the house, forget about it, it's like a small disaster—and almost torture to clean up. But a Yorkie's mistake is almost nothing at all. And that's a good deal in my book, because cleaning the carpet always seems to end up being my job. And one more selling point about this breed, to get my buddies jealous, is that Yorkies do not shed. Not one hair. So, no dog hair on the furniture or on the rug. And no animal dander allergies to worry about either, for you, your kids, or for people coming to visit.

This puppy's new name—Peanut—seemed automatic

because of her size. Jet black when we got her, Peanut's hair quickly turned silvery-blond, a characteristic of her breed. Like Scooter in so many wonderful ways, Peanut has boundless energy and enthusiasm for play. Her lackluster personality when we first got her was directly the result of her being the runt of the litter. Within twenty-four hours of getting a good meal and a good night's sleep (which she had apparently never gotten before because her siblings were always bullying her), Peanut was on top of the world and so ready and willing to run, play ball, and swim in the pond that it seemed like she almost never tired.

And when Peanut first met Rocky, she couldn't believe her eyes. What was this thing? Peanut loves chasing large gray squirrels around our yard, but whenever they slow down, she slows down. She never has and never will catch one, if she continues this technique. But I think she's actually playing with them, anyway—she means them no harm. The gray squirrels seem to know that as well when they intentionally climb down a tree trunk almost to the ground, face-to-face with her. Then they start chattering away at her like there's no tomorrow, Peanut with the most puzzled look on her face, not getting any respect at all.

Peanut doesn't seem to know that Rocky is a squirrel like the gray squirrels she is familiar with. She also doesn't seem to know she's a dog. Like Rocky, we got Peanut so young that she imprinted on Peggy and me, making her identify more with humans than their own species.

This is most evident when Peanut is playing outside with Brian and Christie and the neighborhood kids. Despite her small size, she is always right in the thick of things with the kids. Fearlessly friendly, very alert not to get stepped on, yet right in the middle of every game of soccer, football, baseball, kids' tunneling projects in the dirt, skim boarding on the sandbars at low tide off the dock—if Peggy and I want to know where Peanut is outside, all we have to do is listen for the sound of children, and she'll be right in the middle of them.

Peggy keeps Peanut's hair relatively short, like she did with Scooter. Every couple of weeks, Peggy has her out on our back porch with a set of scissors in her hands, clip-clipping away. Some people let their Yorkies grow their hair out really long, for show. Not us. Peanut is such a hearty little dog, digging in the woods, swimming in the pond, the river, and at the beach like a true water dog, that if she had long hair it would look like a disaster, kind of like the comedian Carrot Top.

Peanut sleeps next to our bed at night. Early every morning, I half awaken, then fall back to sleep. When I wake up for good, an hour or two later, Peanut is asleep, stretched out along my back for warmth, under my arm, between Peggy and me, just like a big dog.

When Peanut finally awakes, she often falls out of bed, then trots over to see Rocky in the corner of the kitchen, now contemplating bedding down for the day in his bungalow full of fluffy white cotton balls. Often they will kiss, nose to nose, then excitedly start chirping and barking at each other, like they just told each other something unbelievable. It's adorable.

Rocky and his roommates. I really got their support when I needed it most. In fact, I probably couldn't have healed so well without all the different animals in our family, including Rocky, Scooter, Peanut, Mitten, Little Rascal and Tex, as well as Peggy, Christie and Brian, my parents, siblings, and friends—in other words, all the bigger animals in my life.

And I'm also forever in debt to the doctors and nurses who cut me up as carefully as possible, then gently put me back together again, so I could get back to the only place on earth where I could truly heal—in our home and in our backyard—with our family, our pets, and the magnificence of Mother Nature.

12

The Discovery of Rocky on Animal Planet and PBS

*N*ot long after my first book came out, I was interviewed by a very talented freelance journalist, Chris Rodell, a rather devout Christian who loved reporting on unusual true-life stories. Evidently mine qualified. The interview resulted in a full-page article in the *National Enquirer* titled "Meet the Luckiest Unlucky Man Alive." This tabloid has one of the largest circulations of any newspaper in the world. The article was so well received that Chris wrote a follow-up five-page story for the notoriously entertaining *Maxim* magazine titled "He Gave Death the Finger 21 Times."

The article was exceedingly funny, accurate, and full of wild color photos. With Lucy Lawless, the actress who played the title role in *Xena: Warrior Princess*, on the cover of the magazine, it was the first issue of *Maxim* to sell over a million copies. At about the same time on the opposite end of the publishing spectrum was another article on my life published in *The Daily Word*, a monthly nondenominational Christian magazine that is distributed by the millions around the world. It was titled, "Yes, God Is Listening."

Both pieces went into great detail about how a thirty-eight-year-old married guy with kids got a deadly form of cancer—probably from the sun—and was told he was going to die. And how, through a combination of early detection, aggressive treatment, the Five Fs, and a whole lot of luck and prayers, he got through the cancer challenge.

I was hoping these articles would help to educate a wide audience about cancer, reaching the far right and left and everyone in between. The wonderful letters and e-mails I received from readers of both publications showed that I was proceeding down the right path. A path to educate people about how to detect cancer at the earliest and most curable stages and then, without delay, to deal with it appropriately.

And, if early detection was not possible, how people could still be helped tremendously, by inspiring and motivating them to do what it takes to raise the quality of their physical and spiritual lives. This could largely be accomplished through the pursuit of greater fulfillment, both at work and at home.

Here's the closing paragraph in the *Daily Word* article:

"If I were told I was going to die tomorrow, I would have no fear. I would have a profound sadness that I was leaving my wife and kids to fend for themselves. Yet I believe God is like the ocean and my life is like an eyedropper full of that ocean. When my life as I know it ends, the eyedropper that is me will go back into the ocean. Then I will instantly explode into all the wonderfulness of God."

Soon, a major milestone was to occur. Peggy and my

dreams and prayers had been answered. Together, we would attend Christie and Brian's sixth-grade graduation. And I'd arrive at the five-year mark cancer-free.

It was a great day. The auditorium at Paterson Elementary was packed full with proud parents and nervous twelve-year-olds. A rousing and very funny speech was given by the principal. And then one by one the names were called off as the children were asked to center stage to receive their graduation diplomas. ". . . Brian William Goss . . . Christina Marie Goss . . ." My eyes watered up and I grabbed hold of Peggy's hand as we sat among the many proud parents.

I knew that most of the parents I was sitting among did not know or understand the challenge that Peggy and I had been through over the past five years. I also knew that there were many challenges that had occurred to the other parents in that room that Peggy and I were completely unaware of. Other people battling cancer, heart disease, diabetes, or a host of other very difficult illnesses. Other people dealing with tragic accidents, or terrible marital turmoil, or depression triggered by great unhappiness at work or at home. I had to force myself into these other people's shoes; even if I didn't know who they were or what they were dealing with, they existed nonetheless. I did not want my present great fortune to blind me to the problems of others.

In my delight at being spared an early death, and in my delight at Peggy and I fulfilling our dream of sitting in the audience, anonymously, watching our two wonderful kids transform from radiant children to glowing young adults, I knew I had been given a gift. A gift I should not take for granted. A gift that, as much as I had worked for it, was still a gift. A gift, that, under different circumstances, could have been taken from me no matter how hard I had tried. I had to remind myself—and I have to do so every day—to be humble—or at least try to be humble.

About six months after I had been diagnosed with cancer, I volunteered to teach self-defense at a nearby shelter for battered women and victims of domestic violence. With a background in boxing, wrestling, football, and always a keen interest in basic self-defense, it was easy to show these women how to break holds and neutralize an opponent. What was not so easy was listening to their stories—so many of them were so heart wrenching. I try to put myself in their shoes. This has helped to humble me. I try to teach at the shelter whenever they ask, because the smile I get from these women after they learn a simple technique to break or neutralize an attack on them, well, this far more than equals what I give them.

And in regard to being humble, if you're old enough to have watched *M*A*S*H*, either the movie or the long-running television show by the same name, you might recall the very shy and humble character Corporal Radar O'Reilly, played by the talented actor Gary Burghoff. Well, PBS called and invited Rocky and the Goss family to do a segment on a show they were putting together called *Pets: Part of the Family*. They did the shoot in our home and backyard. It turned out to be a wonderful piece that PBS routinely broadcasts.

Rocky has stage presence. He's a natural. Every time he's in front of a camera, it stuns me how good he is, like he knows exactly what he's supposed to be doing next. Like he's already thought everything through. Like it's been preordained. Like he's been heaven-sent.

It's a lot of hard work to do these television pieces properly. In a large way, the success of the PBS show had to do with the superior job done by the production team and the host,

Gary Burghoff, a huge animal lover in his own right. Gary Burghoff ended the show with these insightful words:

"For me, Bill's story is a wonderful example of how the bond between a person and an animal can take us into uncharted territory. It reminds me of Norman Cousins, the famous writer who cured himself of cancer by laughing at funny movies. Mysteries don't always have to be explained in the same way that life doesn't have to be completely understood to be enjoyed. I think if our animal friends could speak they might say, 'Don't try to understand us—just enjoy us.' "

After the PBS show aired, the Discovery Channel, which created Animal Planet, called us. They wanted to know whether Rocky would be interested in having his own show—an entire half hour—on Animal Planet. After consulting with Rocky (and Peggy), I returned the call and said yes.

Involving three days of shooting with two talented producers, the always entertaining Tom Baldrick and indefatigable Bud Fraga, it was a real learning experience for me from start to finish.

The first third of the show was shot in our backyard and the second third in our kitchen. Again, Rocky performed flawlessly, as if on cue. The cameraman used a tiny lipstick camera to get great close-ups of Rocky in his little white house as well as in my shirt pocket. The Animal Planet production crew then traveled with me as I went to give a speech to a local group of retired businessmen. During the speech, Rocky routinely jumped from my head to my shoulder, then into my pocket and back out again. Then, back at the house again, they shot footage of me cleaning Rocky's cage while I explained the care and feeding of flying squirrels in general.

In the last part of the show, I ended up taking Rocky flying over northeastern Florida in an ultralight airplane owned by my friend Gary La Pierre. Rocky was in the top left pocket of my old Navy flight suit. Little remote-control-operated lipstick cameras were taped to various spots in the cockpit to capture the spirit of the moment. Rocky seemed to love the whole experience.

It turned out to be a wonderfully inspiring and uplifting half-hour episode, titled *Rocky the Flying Squirrel*, part of the series called *Pet Stories* that airs on Animal Planet. Translated into several languages, the show is routinely transmitted by satellite into many millions of homes around the world. If you want to see when it's going to be broadcast again, just visit my web site: www. BillGoss.com.

Immediately after the show was broadcast on Animal Planet, I got a call from a woman in New York City named Freya Manston. A tremendous animal lover, particularly of cats, she explained how she'd been involved in the publishing business for most of her life. Freya had been Danielle Steele's first editor, and then later, as a literary agent, she represented Katharine Hepburn for her intriguing autobiography, *Me*.

Freya had seen the Animal Planet show and loved it. After some small talk, Freya asked if I wanted a New York–based literary agent to represent me.

I said yes. Gladly.

13

Life Is Good

Freya was good to her word. She said she could get me a book deal with a major New York publishing house, and in relatively short order she did just that, using the opening chapter of this book and a three-page chapter outline.

Now, with a signed contract in my hand, all I had to do was to sit down and write the sucker. No easy task.

Writing an autobiographical book like this can be kind of tricky, because you're living the story while you're writing it. Not only are there some crazy biases that are automatically built in to autobiographical works, but there are things I might think significant about Rocky and cancer and my life that my editors think are boring, inappropriate, or even gross. Thankfully, this doesn't happen too often.

And also, since none of this stuff is make-believe, sometimes you have to wait for tomorrow to happen before you can continue writing something that is worthy of someone's time and effort—yours, specifically—to read.

Often, as a writer, I feel obliged to share my fears with you, and that can be uncomfortable, not only for me but for my wife and other family members as well, because of the highly personal nature of it all.

And in this regard, I've got to tell you—I've still had some scares related to cancer, even years later.

Like after the first airing of the Animal Planet show, Peggy, Christie, Brian, and I took a trip into the Great Smokies. Within this trip, Brian had planned out a two-day father-son adventure where he and I would do a particularly rigorous hike back and forth along the fifteen highest miles of the Appalachian Trail. The plan was for Peggy and Christie to stay in a hotel in Gatlinburg, Tennessee, and then hook up with us again after Brian and I returned from the mountains.

At 6,500 feet, right along the mountain's crest that separates Tennessee from North Carolina, it was as beautiful as you can imagine, but very tough hiking. After going deep into the wilderness for about ten miles, Brian and I, completely tuckered out, relaxed on a sunny grassy knoll near a spring, a place with a tremendously expansive view of the Great Smokies. Getting really comfortable, too comfortable in fact, we decided to pitch a tent and spend the night at this gorgeous mountaintop retreat.

Fortunately (from an adventure aspect) and unfortunately (because it scared the daylights out of us) we woke up with a large black bear right in our faces and decided it was time to head back to civilization. Brian's comment on our hike out said it all: "Dad, I really wanted to see a bear close up on this trip—but not *that* close."

Shortly after that trip, I started feeling really lousy. I thought it might have been caused by drinking from a crystal-clear spring high on the mountain. But I tested negative for anything caused by impure water. (Which I viewed as bad news, not good—I was hoping it was only something so simple as that.) Soon I was feeling weak and tired all the time, with a very minor rash over my right eye and a bad headache. What was scaring me most was that I was starting to lose my excellent vision—rapidly. Every day, my vision was becoming more and more blurred.

Of course, I became very concerned that melanoma tumors had metastasized from my left ear into my brain. "Brain mets," as they are called by doctors, was not an illogical conclusion by any stretch of the imagination. It had happened to two people I knew over the past couple of years and had killed both of them. And my doctor agreed that this was certainly a possibility.

If this was happening to me, I wanted to know about it as soon as possible, because the earlier the better is always the rule with cancer. *Always.*

Never even remotely a hypochondriac before cancer, it bothered me that after cancer, I was forced to become something of a worrywart about seemingly minor illnesses. But—I was cautioned by my doctors—if I wanted to stay alive for a long time, I would have to listen and be sensitive to my body more than ever before. I'd have to investigate carefully anything I was feeling or sensing that was different from normal if I wanted a shot at living a long and healthy life.

Because of the headaches and rapid loss of visual acuity, my doctor scheduled me for an MRI. Magnetic resonance imaging is often recommended over CAT scans in determining soft-tissue disorders of the brain caused by cancer.

At the MRI facility, I was placed in a prone position within a magnetic coil, and radio-frequency energy was applied to my body. The radio waves excited the protons that form the nuclei of the trillions of hydrogen atoms within my body. This was then used to construct a computer image of the soft tissues of my brain. (According to my closest friends—very soft tissue.)

Since MRI hardly visualizes bone, it provides especially good images of the contents of the skull and spinal column.

A few days later, my MRI results came back. Normal—negative for cancer—greatly reducing the stress around the Goss household. With the knowledge that it was not cancer, I was able to wait much more patiently, hoping I would start feeling better on my own, something not possible to do with a diagnosis of metastatic cancer. Within two months, powered by my body's immune system, and my family and Rocky's comfort and support, I came to feel completely better. Thankfully, my vision returned to normal—better than 20/20.

One of my doctors now believes I had an unusual case of shingles, a nerve disorder related to the chicken pox virus, which lies dormant within most adults. For most adults (children often get chicken pox but rarely get shingles), this nerve disorder seems to come from out of nowhere—but doctors theorize that it usually is induced by stress. My doctor's diagnosis of shingles also explained the rash over my right eye, a frequent symptom, except these rashes almost always cause great pain. I had experienced a dull throbbing headache but none of the extreme pain usually associated with this not uncommon flare-up of nerves.

After recovering, for about a year I felt terrific. Then, for the second time, I developed some significant swelling of the lymph nodes in my armpits, often referred to by doctors as the axial nodes. With the swollen axial nodes—and after having learned that skin cancers like malignant melanoma take approximately one life every hour of every day—I again sought out professional advice.

My superb dermatologists, Dr. Barbara Ebert and Dr. George Schmeider, completely understood my concerns and suggested I get a PET (positron emission tomography) scan.

Newer technology than CAT scans and MRIs, the PET scan is an excellent diagnostic tool for detecting areas of abnormally high metabolic and biochemical activity (typically caused by higher than normal glucose uptake). This kind of activity in your body is usually associated with fast-growing cancer cells.

PET scans are excellent for detecting metastatic melanoma, a tumor known for its high degree of metabolic activity relative to the surrounding tissue in which it is imbedded. PET uses specialized computer imaging equipment and rings of detectors around you to record the gamma radiation produced when the positrons (positively charged particles) emitted by the radioactive tracer—it's injected into your bloodstream before your scan begins—collide with electrons.

Usually, data from your PET scan is evaluated against a separate CAT scan by a radiologist to attain an accurate comparative diagnosis. One piece of equipment has been designed to do PET and CAT scans simultaneously, though I don't know what they're calling it.

Thankfully, after the radiology department compared my PET scan with my CAT scan, I was again determined cancer-free. And now, at the seven-year cancer-free mark, with such high-quality technology looking into my body and finding nothing, I felt I could start to breathe much easier about any new aches and pains I had.

So, with science to back me up, I moved forward again, finally cut free from the constraints of wondering what was going on inside my body, thanks to the latest and greatest in cutting-edge technologies.

New imaging technologies, and the companies that are making these available to all of us, are changing the face of personalized health care, allowing people like you and me to move forward with our lives, confident we're staying ahead of the disease curve. What is available to us now and what will be available to us in the future is mind-boggling. Because of these new medical technologies, people around the world will be living longer, healthier, happier, and more fulfilled lives—guaranteed.

With renewed confidence in my health, I traveled to New Hampshire to give an inspirational keynote speech to the top Century 21 office in New England. The founder and owner of this particular real-estate office is another life-long friend, Jim "Jungle James" Mardis. An amazingly entrepreneurial guy, Jim worked part-time clearing brush for a builder while attending college in New Hampsire. Jim somehow came to the conclusion that successful high-technology business people would generate a huge demand for vacation homes. He felt they would particularly want waterfront properties on the enormous Lake Winnipesaukee in central New Hampshire. Jim and I had hiked and camped all over New Jersey, New Hampshire, and Massachusetts during our spring and summer breaks at Millburn High School. But obviously, while I was goofing off during our many misadventures together, Jim must have been doing informal demographics.

On my return, Rocky and I were invited to attend Jacksonville's annual Fur Ball, a major black-tie affair in northeastern Florida. Let me explain. It's a formal affair in which people bring their pets with them, dressed in formal wear if possible. The more colorful the outfits on the dogs and cats and pot-belled pigs, the better. Chihuahuas in tutus. Bulldogs in tuxedos. Cats in evening gowns. But an internationally known flying squirrel by the name of Rocky had never attended such an event before.

Rocky rode around on my shoulder, perfectly at ease with the hundreds of dressed-up dogs, cats, birds, pigs, and many other animals. This delightful annual event, organized by many people, including my friends Pat, Kelly, and Seana Delaney, was a big success that raised a lot of money for the Jacksonville Humane Society, in existence since 1885. The money raised at the Fur Ball helped pay for the care of the fourteen thousand unwanted and abused animals coming through their doors each year.

I also started doing some extensive business consulting for companies in the fields of media relations, corporate fund-raising, and strategic relationship building. One company generously sent me to the Harvard Business School's Executive Education Program. As I sat in class in Cambridge, in one of the world's most renowned institutes of higher learning, I thought to myself, This isn't half bad—especially for a former garbage man from New Jersey. . . . But seriously speaking, attending that course at Harvard was an incredible experience—one that I will always treasure, particularly because of the friendships I developed with some of the professors. Harvard Business School even ended up using a quote from me in one of their course brochures.

During another consulting engagement, Jeff Marcketta and I, along with two other businesspeople, attended the Masters Tournament in Augusta, Georgia. I copiloted the plane both up and back. The aircraft was similar to the type in which I had been a senior flight instructor when Peggy and I lived in Texas.

While at the Masters, we had the opportunity to briefly

meet Tiger Woods, and later, the four of us were invited into the historic Green Jacket Club as personal guests of Arnold Palmer for refreshments while a thunderstorm passed overhead. While consulting, speaking, and writing, you can end up in all kinds of unusual places and situations.

The Young Entrepreneur Organization in Silicon Valley recently asked me to speak. With one hundred chapters and five thousand members, this is a large and well-organized group loaded up with some of America's brightest young business stars. I was to be accompanied at this talk by my loyal buddy Jamis McNiven, the owner-founder of Buck's Restaurant in Woodside, California. Jamis is a masterful impresario and entrepreneur unlike any other in the world. Before he opened Buck's, Jamis was a builder. A builder with unusual clients. He and his close friend Josh Shade built a huge home for the founder of Apple Computer, Steven Jobs. Jamis also built the first Planet Hollywood.

One of the things Buck's Restaurant is famous for is the gigantic hand-carved twenty-foot-long fish—actually a salmon, according to Jamis—parked on the street directly in front of the restaurant. Many entrepreneurial plans were first presented to venture-capital firms at Buck's—often drafted on the restaurant's napkins. Companies such as Netscape, Hotmail, and Yahoo, to name just a few. With the ups and downs of the stock market, I don't know whether this was necessarily a good thing or not, but I can guarantee you this—the food there is always good, especially Jamis's world-famous (in Woodside) pumpkin pancakes.

To be a member of the Young Entrepreneurs, you have to be under forty and have started a multimillion-dollar company. I think they wanted Jamis and me to speak mainly for the laughs. Since Jamis is widely referred to as the Prime Minister of Silicon Valley, and my expertise is in survival, resilience, and fulfillment, I'm sure we'll be able to deliver a worthwhile message to this group of brilliant millionaires (like these people really need our advice!).

Jamis McNiven and his family are tremendous animal lovers. "Our backyard has Brahman bulls, camels, zebras, emus, peacocks—and even a couple of horses—but nobody pays any attention to them," quipped Jamis. Buck's Restaurant is also famous for its unusual fare. After visiting the McNiven menagerie, you wonder if some of it's homegrown.

Besides business consulting, I started doing consulting directly related to cancer research. Funded by the National Institutes of Health (NIH), the National Cancer Institute hired me as a patient-advocate consultant for my expertise in various aspects of skin cancers, particularly malignant melanoma. This is intriguing work because it puts me in direct contact with some of the world's leading doctors, specialists with M.D. and/or Ph.D. degrees in broad areas of cancer research.

One of the large NIH/NCI programs I'm involved with is SPORE (Selected Programs of Research Excellence), where we meet to help decide funding of future cancer research in a wide array of projects.

This consulting work is usually conducted in Washington, D.C. But it has involved other institutions as well, such as the University of Texas M.D. Anderson Cancer Center and Duke University Medical Center.

Some of these research studies may be familiar to you, such as *angiogenesis,* which is when there is an increase in the formation of blood vessels to feed a rapidly growing tumor. Preventing angiogenesis should prevent cancerous tumors from growing and spreading at such a rapid rate.

Apoptosis, which is programmed cell death, is a healthy,

normal, and naturally occurring cellular process that shuts off for some reason in cancer cells, allowing them to grow out of control, like a wildfire. Inducing apoptosis—making cells die after fifty to one hundred divisions, like most of the body's other cells—is another unique strategy that may ultimately prove to be a cure for cancer.

There are many other interesting studies regarding cancer and hormone levels (estrogen, testosterone, DHEA, etc.) as well as *gene therapy*. One involves a virus believed to be harmless to humans, but it's loaded with a gene inside called p53 that normally suppresses tumors. In many cancer patients, the p53 gene appears to be defective. Introducing the virus into animals with cancer appears to zero in on that flaw, by harming the cancer cells but leaving the normal healthy cells unscathed. Using rodent studies (except for Rocky, it's still a bad time to be a rodent), researchers injected this virus into mice with existing colon cancer. The results were extremely significant, eliminating tumors in six of the ten animals.

I attended several extremely comprehensive seminars on breast and ovarian cancer conducted by some of the leading medical researchers in the world. One thing I learned that came as a surprise to me was that for every one hundred people with breast cancer, one of them is a man.

At a seminar on prostate cancer, I learned from a urologist that one of his patients had a PSA (prostate specific antigen) reading of over 26,000. Frankly, since a psa reading over four is considered a red flag by many doctors, I had no idea a PSA level could go so high.

The National Institutes of Health and the National Cancer Institute found out about me via the medical newsletters and magazines I've been asked to write for, such as the Memorial

Sloan-Kettering Melanoma Update, the American Melanoma Foundation (a wonderful organization whose web site links to BillGoss.com), The Cancer Club (CancerClub.com) and *Coping with Cancer* magazine.

The same week I was in Washington consulting for the NIH—and also visiting my old Navy buddy Frank Gren, at Galway Partners—I was invited to attend a weekend reunion in Canada, on an incredible little island in the middle of the St. Lawrence Seaway. This get-together was comprised of eight of my close buddies from the township of Millburn-Short Hills, New Jersey. Some of us had attended kindergarten, grade school, and junior and senior high school together. Talk about a brotherhood of men. Throughout those formative years, we spent tremendous amounts of time together in various heavily wooded areas of New Jersey—hiking, camping, fishing, bird-watching, swimming, snake hunting—sometimes with our girlfriends, sometimes without. But always—and I mean always—we had an absolutely great time together. That was guaranteed.

For this reunion, we were going to a place where we could relive many of those good times. Yet, instead of being six or sixteen years old, now we were forty-six. In the blink of an eye, we had gone from being babies to baby boomers.

What a fun and wild and woolly trip it turned out to be. We were hosted by the unsinkable Flory and Joan Bastile, the in-laws of Mike "Chelsea" McCollough. With his uncanny persuasive abilities, Chelsea had somehow convinced Flory and Joan to entrust "the men" with their gorgeous little two-story cabin, and their watercraft, and their well-stocked outdoor bar—aptly nicknamed the Red Fin Lounge for the type of fish that spawned each year in the creek right next to the cabin.

Flory had owned several restaurants, and boy, does this man know how to entertain and feed people. The food was unbelievable. Greg "Rat" O'Neil picked me up at the airport in Syracuse, New York, and we drove two hours north to the U.S.–Canadian border. Rat, in his inimitable way, almost got us thrown out of Canada before we even got in. Finally making it across the border, we were met by Chris "Cubie" McHugh, John "Grimmer" Grimm, Carl "Gureenie" Guarino, Dick "Wildman" Crowley, Mark "Fuzz" Landis, and Jon "Killer" Kilik.

We went fishing for smallmouth bass, pike, and muskie (huge predator fish that look like immense sixty-pound pike on steroids). And we did our annual cliff jumping into the river (we'd finally wised up and no longer dove headfirst) and generally tooled around on a pontoon boat together enjoying the great outdoors. It was some real quality male-bonding time. Everybody ought to do this now and then, I thought to myself, as I watched the sun set over the shimmering river with some of my best buddies.

The following morning, after the worst late-night karaoke competition you've ever heard, we all came to the conclusion that although forty years had passed since some of us had first met, we really hadn't changed that much, except for the additional growth of hair on our backs and the reduction of it on our heads. And our voices were far worse for the wear. I actually think that bats, barn swallows, and other creatures of the night sky fell to earth, paralyzed, so awful was our singing. But we sang on, immensely enjoying being out in the woods together, laughing it up by a huge, blazing campfire underneath an immense starlit sky, and swimming in the ice-cold water of the St. Lawrence River.

I reflected on my Five Fs of Fulfillment: Family, Friends, Faith, Focus and Fun. This had been a serious dose of Friends and Fun. Every one of us left with a new and revitalized human spirit, ready to face the rat race again. No matter how hard it sometimes seemed that the world wanted to hit us right between the eyes, we were ready to dive back into it again, with gusto.

Back from that thoroughly invigorating trip, I flew out to Houston to visit with another friend, Kevin Saunders, at a time when he was being considered as a potential candidate to be the next chairman of the President's Council on Physical Fitness and Sports (PCPF&S), a board he sat on during the Bush and the Clinton administrations. His story is a totally remarkable one, because he, too, fell to earth like Rocky, but Kevin's landing was a whole lot harder.

I met Kevin when we were both giving motivational speeches in the same hotel. Kevin, a paraplegic, is considered one of the finest wheelchair athletes in the world. As Kevin and I talked and became familiar with each other, we learned something remarkable about the strange world of coincidence, happenstance, and serendipity.

Years ago, I was a Navy student pilot flying a practice instrument approach into Corpus Christi International Airport at about one thousand feet and descending rapidly. All of a sudden the instructor took the aircraft from me and said, "Oh my God—Ensign Goss, take a look down there!" He wrapped the airplane into a hard ninety-degree angle of bank turn, standing the airplane virtually on its wingtip, allowing me to look straight down at the ground. Directly below us, explosions were going off. Big explosions with lots of fire. One of the world's tallest grain elevators was blowing up.

Kevin, in his midtwenties at the time, like myself, was also flying through the air at that moment. But his flight below me lasted at only three hundred feet—and it was without an airplane.

Kevin had just been inspecting the giant grain elevator for explosive grain dust and discovered it contained the dust at dangerous levels. Before he could get the problem corrected: *kaboom!* It blew up in a fiery explosion that left ten people dead and another thirty seriously injured. Kevin landed in a parking lot three hundred feet from where he'd first felt the devastating explosion. He was discovered bent over backward—the wrong way—almost in half, paralyzed from the chest down, with many other terrible injuries and very little blood left. Doctors did not expect him to survive the night.

But, like Christopher Reeve (with whom I've also been blessed to have had a private meeting), the doctors didn't fully comprehend the power of Kevin's unbelievable will to live. And years later he was throwing a shot put, discus, and javelin farther, while sitting in a wheelchair, than they'd ever been thrown before.

As the first member of the PCPF&S with a disability, Kevin helped to educate the American people about how essential the role of physical fitness, sports, and proper nutrition is if you want to have a balanced and fulfilling life—even if you are in a wheelchair.

And speaking of a fulfilling life, there is one thing that Rocky hasn't done yet that I think would really round out his life. It's time for him to become a father. Peggy, Christie, and Brian agreed. We needed a female flying squirrel, a Rockette, if you will, to bring Rocky's life full circle.

So on the Internet I went, typing "Flying Squirrels" into Netscape's search engine. Bang—in the blink of an eye I had a plethora of information at my fingertips. I ended up buying a wonderful little book about the care and husbandry of southern flying squirrels written by the late Curt Howard, the leading expert on the subject. If you go to BillGoss.com, you'll see a link directly to one of the flying squirrel web sites inspired by Curt.

The flying squirrel parts of this book are, in a way, a memorial to Curt Howard. Why? Because early one morning he died in a car accident, just after delivering a baby flying squirrel to a person in need. In need of a little angel. Curt, along with his wife, Judy, had personally bred and raised thousands of southern flying squirrels throughout the years. Curt taught me more about how to enrich and extend Rocky's life than any other person on the planet. If there is a God—and I believe there is, with all my heart—then Curt's not only soaring with the angels, he's soaring with the flying squirrels.

I asked Judy to put Peggy and me on the waiting list for a new baby—a baby female flying squirrel, that is. After we get our little Rockette, it's estimated it will take a year of dating before Rocky and his little Rockette start a family. We hope they'll create a Rocky Two, Three, Four, and so forth, just like Sylvester Stallone did. Maybe they'll be able to provide us with a whole team of dancing Rockettes as well.

The Rock is getting older, so I hope he still has it in him, if you know what I mean. I think he does. I hope he does. Only time will tell. Next year, I'll write another book about how the Rock and Rockette fell in love and started a family, if you want me to do that for you.

Why not now? Why not in this book? Because this book is going to end the same way it started. Flying fast. Really fast. I opened chapter one by going Mach one. I figured it would be appropriate to close the final chapter by going Mach two. Actually, I didn't dream up this idea. A friend of mine, Jennifer Carroll, who worked for the same dynamic Navy admiral I did, Kevin Delaney, set the whole thing up.

Jennifer, a mustang like myself, was born in Trinidad and raised in New York City, where she enlisted in the U.S. Navy as a jet mechanic. Rapidly rising through the ranks, she retired as a lieutenant commander, then ran for a seat in the U.S. Congress. She lost the first time, but I'm willing to bet she'll win next time. Because, like my friend Rudy Ruettiger from the movie *Rudy*, Jennifer does not give up, and I am completely convinced that persistence *always* pays off.

Now, as the executive director of Florida's Department of Veterans Affairs, Jennifer thought a retired military baby boomer going Mach two—and then writing about it—would be a marvelous way to show the world that veterans, individually and as a group, are very much alive and kicking.

So, the day after Jennifer and I talked, I got a call from General Doug Burnett, the senior officer in charge of the Florida Air National Guard. Jennifer had called him and he liked the idea. He figured it would be a great way to promote the Air National Guard as well, an incredible organization that my son, Brian, has already starting talking about.

The mission of the Air National Guard is primarily homeland defense. Not an easy task when you consider the fact that the United States of America has 20,000 miles of borders. Or that it has 600,000 bridges, 170,000 water systems, around 3,000 power plants (104 that are nuclear), hundreds of thousands of miles of natural-gas pipelines and train tracks, around 500 skyscrapers taller than 500 feet, and countless sports stadiums, airports, schools, and large public and corporate structures. It's all part of the infrastructure behind this nation of nearly 300 million people spread out over 3.7 million square miles.

Defense of the homeland is a huge undertaking, but one that the Air National Guard, National Guard, Coast Guard, Navy, Marines, Air Force, and Army—all the men and women in the armed services—stand ready to do, especially when the will of the American people is behind them.

But regarding my orientation flight with the Air National Guard, part of the deal was that Rocky, the world's smallest aviator, would have to come visit with some of General Burnett's biggest and brightest top guns, the aviators and the support people of the Florida Air National Guard.

For some reason, it seems that military people, in particular, get a kick out of flying squirrels. Even one of our former commanders in chief, President Teddy Roosevelt, the famous leader of the supermacho Rough Riders, had a pet flying squirrel. He found them irresistibly cute, entertaining, and always able to generate a belly laugh.

Apparently no president had more animals in the White House than Roosevelt. One story the President liked sharing with people was how his bull terrier, Pete, had torn the pants off the new ambassador to France. As soon as the ambassador somehow got his pants back on, Roosevelt's pet flying squirrel, from seemingly out of nowhere, landed on the poor guy's shoulder and nearly gave him a heart attack. Roosevelt thought the whole thing was hilarious.

The earliest known writings about flying squirrels were in 1606 by Captain John Smith, governor of the Johnstown colony. He wrote how the local Indians kept as pets "a small beast they call Assapanick, but we call them flying squirrels, because by spreading their legs, and so stretching the largeness of their skins, they have been seen to fly 30 to 40 yards."

So, as I explained to General Burnett, flying squirrels have a long history involved with the military and the leading members of the U.S. government. But, most of all, I knew why General Burnett would like Rocky—because, like himself, Rocky was an aviator.

While waiting for my F-15 Eagle flight with the Florida Air National Guard, I continued writing in my home office. Life is good. Always choose life.

14

The Attack on America and the Supercharging of the Human Spirit

We must take a stand against terrorism in the world and combat it with firmness, for it is a most cowardly and savage violation of peace. We must remember our heritage, who we are and what we are, and how this nation, this island of freedom, came into being. And we must make it unmistakably plain to all the world that we have no intention of compromising our principles, our beliefs, or our freedom, that we have the will and the determination to do as a young president, John Kennedy, said in his inaugural address: "Bear any burden, pay any price."

—RONALD REAGAN

A few days after accepting General Burnett's generous invitation to receive an orientation flight in one of the Florida
Air National Guard's F-15 Eagles, the world suddenly accelerated to hypersonic speed.

Then, in the mere blink of an eye, my Mach two flight was
postponed—and the world as we knew it was instantly turned
upside down.

I'm sure you'll never forget where you were or what you
were doing when it happened. Like when President Kennedy
was assassinated—I was playing marbles in the dirt in front of
Wyoming Elementary School and suddenly I heard a teacher
cry out to another teacher, "Oh my God, the President's been
shot—oh my God—the President's been shot!"

I was in my office at home writing this book. The phone
rang. It was Eli Silberman, a dear friend and business associate
from Pennsylvania. He asked me if I knew what was going on. I
didn't know what he was talking about. Then he told me to
turn on the television.

There, on every channel, I saw a familiar sight, the twin
towers of the World Trade Center, on the southern tip of
Manhattan, the Big Apple. Rocky and I had looked down at
them when we flew in to do *Sally Jessy Raphael* together. Now,
right before my eyes and on every channel on live TV, I could
see the upper part of the North Tower completely ablaze. Eli, a
former U.S. Marine officer, told me how he thought America
was under attack, and I listened to him in complete disbelief as
together we watched a second airliner, this one a United States
Boeing 767 loaded with people and fuel, originally en route
from Boston to Los Angeles, slam into the South Tower.

It was Tuesday, September 11, 2001, at 9:03 A.M.

We—Eli in Pennsylvania, myself in Florida—then watched

in horror as people jumped for their lives to escape the flames. It seemed like a Hollywood movie, it just could not be real. It just was not possible. Like being told I had cancer—I was in a state of complete denial. I had to be dreaming.

Right before our eyes, on live TV, Eli and I watched first the South Tower of the World Trade Center, all 110 floors, then the North Tower of the World Trade Center, all 110 floors, collapse straight down, completely to the ground. Never before had I witnessed anything of such magnitude.

Then Dan Rather told us that an American Airlines 757 had just crashed into the side of the Pentagon. Moments later he told us a United Airlines 757 had crashed in a wooded area of western Pennsylvania.

In the space of less than two hours, four of America's most modern passenger jets had been hijacked and systematically turned into suicide bombs. Close to 3000 innocent people of various nationalities and religions were killed by a radical fundamentalist religious terrorist organization. Nearly 3000 people no longer with us in physical body, but who will be forever with us in our hearts and souls. Still vitally alive, because the human spirit does not and cannot die, only the physical body.

And the symbol of that human spirit could be seen in the foreground of the smoking ruins of the World Trade Center towers—standing tall, holding high the torch of freedom, the Statue of Liberty. Holding high the torch whose meaning the terrorists tried so hard to extinguish—freedom's flame. Liberty's flame. This same flame will light up and remove the darkness of terrorism if we no longer take this great symbol for granted, but look at it for what it is, a symbol for freedom-loving people everywhere, a symbol in direct opposition to what world terrorism represents—slavery and domination of the human spirit, especially that of women and children.

(These terrorists had been both jealous of and wondering how North America and modern society in general had surged ahead of them over the course of history. Perhaps it was because they have denied themselves of the talents, imagination, and energy of half their population—the women.)

The only crime the innocent victims committed was to show up at work or at the airport on time. Good and wonderful people whose lives were ended by bad people.

The attack against America, according to the terrorists, was committed in the name of God. It's hard to imagine how anyone could possibly think that an all-merciful and loving God would want us to intentionally murder innocent people, but that is what the terrorists would have us believe.

I had close friends in both the World Trade Center and the Pentagon. Thankfully—and very luckily—they survived. A friend from Millburn High School, Michael Simoff, sent me this e-mail:

"Bill, I was in the building right across the street and saw it happen, 300 feet west and they would have gotten me. I'm so glad to be alive."

Other people I know weren't so fortunate. My high school football coach, Matt Sellitto, lost his son, Matthew, age twenty-three, a wonderful young man just getting started in life. He worked for Cantor Fitzgerald, a firm that lost nearly seven hundred of its one thousand employees in the attack. The McHugh family, very close lifelong friends of mine, lost their first cousin. Both he and Matthew Sellitto were trapped near the top of one of the towers.

Three former Navy P-3 Orion officers were killed in the attack on the Pentagon, two pilots and one flight officer, all of them highly regarded professionals and warm and caring individuals.

One of them, Captain Jack Punches, had been a talented

and kind flight instructor to me when I was a new pilot, learning how to fly the P-3 Orion surveillance aircraft and simultaneously operate its extremely sophisticated electronic systems for the very first time.

One of my closest Navy friends, whom I referred to as "Bo" Mills in my first book, *The Luckiest Unlucky Man Alive*, was working directly for Donald Rumsfeld, the secretary of defense, when American Flight 77 crashed into the west side of the Pentagon. This is what Captain Pat Mills had to say about that experience:

"It felt like a sonic boom from a jet breaking the sound barrier directly overhead. The building shuddered, the windows rattled, and that was it. Soon the air was filled with a pungent smell, like burning wires in an electrical fire. I have to tell you something, Bill. You would have been so proud if you had witnessed with your own eyes the way so many young men and women in uniform responded to this incredible crisis with great courage, honor, and commitment. I only hope our country will consider national defense a top priority now—without it you can forget everything else."

Captain Mills developed the highest admiration for his boss, former college wrestler and Navy pilot Donald Rumsfeld, especially after Pat witnessed him in action. A quote from *The Wall Street Journal*, written on the eve of the new year following the attack, helps clarify what Captain Mills personally observed that day to make him so loyal to the man.

> On the morning the Pentagon was attacked, Mr. Rumsfeld gave the nation a clear display of his own courage and character. He was in the building when the plane hit. He rushed toward the flames to help the injured, only returning to his office to join the

White House in crisis management. That same evening, Sept. 11, Mr. Rumsfeld held the first of these wartime press briefings—in the still burning Pentagon. He launched right into an opening statement about the tragedy, then interrupted himself in the middle of the first sentence to add, "First of all, good evening." It was a minor grace note, but it was also classic Rumsfeld, invoking a world in which the priority would not be to flail and emote and self-promote, but to get a grip and actually deal with the problem. Mr. Rumsfeld went on to assure the country that "the Pentagon's functioning. It will be in business tomorrow."

Working at his desk almost at ground zero at the Pentagon, another Navy friend of mine, Captain Tim Tibbits, shared with me what he experienced that day:

"Bill, the 757 struck the building directly beneath me. There was a tremendous explosion and a huge fireball blew right past my window. While being evacuated through the smoky center courtyard, I saw a piece of an airplane wing lying on the ground. That's when I first knew we had been struck by an airplane just like the twin towers less than an hour earlier. Once outside, we started carrying the wounded to the triage stations that remarkably were in place in less than fifteen minutes. I thank God more people in my office weren't hurt or killed."

Amazingly, many of the terrorist suicide pilots learned to fly right here in our own backyard, trained in American flight schools in Florida and other states.

In almost the blink of an eye, the President, as commander in chief, along with his extremely seasoned cabinet members, took charge. Watching the president speak to the American people on TV, sitting next to Peggy—with Peanut on her lap and Rocky on my shoulder—I felt so damn proud of America it brought tears to my eyes. It inspired me to want to serve this great country all over again. And so, a few days later—as soon as they started accepting applications—I applied for a position as a federal air marshal. Never again did I want to hear of terrorists with box cutters and pocket knives holding airborne Americans hostage. Never again.

With gratitude, I realized that the terrorists had accomplished the exact opposite of what they had hoped to accomplish. They had hoped to break the will of Americans and freedom-loving people everywhere. Instead, they galvanized our will, gave it strength, focus, and resolve. The terrorists, without meaning to, supercharged our human spirit, both as individuals and as a nation. They could not have made a greater error in judgment.

Three generations earlier, after reluctantly executing the surprise attack on Pearl Harbor that suddenly embroiled the United States into WW II, the renown Japanese naval aviator Admiral Yamamoto wondered about the same possibility when he said, "A sleeping giant has been awakened."

Seven years ago, I discovered a small and questionable element in my body. I insisted it be cut out and biopsied. It was a malignant tumor—virtually guaranteed to infiltrate the millions of healthy and normal cells around it. Virtually guaranteed to kill me if I ignored it.

The malignant growth had started as an extremely small and undetectable tumor many years before I first discovered it. How did it start? I don't know. Maybe a bad sunburn when I was a child. To me, the reason was no longer important—I no longer cared, it was superfluous. To me, what was important was only one thing—the cure.

Like cancer, world terrorism had started infiltrating freedom-loving societies like America years ago. At around the same time as the bump on my ear showed up in my life, world terrorism showed up in America. It reared its ugly head with the garage-basement bombing of the World Trade Center. Five people were killed and one thousand injured. Unfortunately, we chose to ignore terrorism's highly malignant qualities. We merely put a Band-Aid on the problem, rather than perform the radical and massive surgery that was required at the time.

In *The Gathering Storm*, Winston Churchill wrote: "If you will not fight for the right, when your victory will be sure and not too costly, you may come to the moment when you will have to fight with all odds against you and only a precarious chance of survival."

This war against terrorism will not be like any other war we've fought. Like fighting cancer, you have to kill all of the bad cells. And, unfortunately—like cancer treatments—some of the good cells will be killed in the process. Innocent people will tragically be killed, but we must stand behind our military and our leadership nonetheless.

And now—with the passage of time that allows all malignancies to dramatically magnify themselves—to overcome world terrorism we will need far greater resources to cure ourselves. Resources in technology, human and financial capital, and national will.

But, just like I believe that if we supercharge our human spirit, we can supercharge our immune systems to fight malignant tumors and other serious illnesses, I believe that if we supercharge our will as freedom-loving people, we will someday—someday soon—eliminate world terrorism just like we will someday—someday soon—eliminate cancer.

Ultimately we will do this by tapping in to our roots, in to our "can do" pioneer spirit and our love and appreciation of the great outdoors. Each and every day, we should tap in to God and country and Mother Nature. We should use them as a reminder that one of our greatest treasures is our freedom to enjoy these things.

But we should also be reminded that far too often there are insidious elements, just like a cancer, that want to rob us of our freedom. Our freedom to enjoy God and our freedom to explore and celebrate the natural beauty of our homeland from sea to shining sea—freedoms that so many of us, myself included, have taken for granted.

We can't ignore the fact that freedom-loving people will always have enemies. And we can't worry solely about terrorist threats in the future. In fact, we must insist upon and be willing to pay for a wide range of security capabilities for the simple reason that our first obligation is to protect ourselves, our families, and our homeland.

Like a pilot flying through congested airspace, we must keep our heads on a swivel, enjoying our unique and blessed view of God's spectacular creativity, but ever vigilant for trouble headed our way. Liberty requires vigilance.

So enjoy your family and friends. Celebrate your faith. Focus on everything that is good but ignore nothing that is bad, and take appropriate action expeditiously and without delay.

And have fun—lots of fun—laughing every day, exercising your sense of humor just like you should exercise your body. Enjoy life and encourage and help others to do the same. Generously love the people and the pets in your life.

According to Dr. Carl Charnetski—a world-renowned professor of psychology—stroking a pet, taking a walk in the woods, loving your spouse, and other things that calm us naturally, significantly boost the release of immunity-enhancing chemicals in our bodies, sometimes by 30 percent or more than when we don't find the time to do these simple little things. Don't forget to revel in the natural beauty and splendid complexity of everything Mother Nature has laid before you.

And keep your eyes open. Especially when you take that walk in the woods I expect you to be doing regularly now—keeping your eyes open for that tiny little ball of fur, your future copilot, that could be falling from the heavens at any moment—like an angel from above—right into your pocket and into your life.

Epilogue

*A*s this book was going to press, Rocky's fiancée blew into town. She came in on a Continental Airlines flight from Houston, where she was born seven weeks earlier at the home of Judy Howard, now one of the top experts in the world on the care and husbandry of southern flying squirrels.

Absolutely adorable, the little female flying squirrel crawled immediately from my hands into my shirt pocket and fell asleep during our drive home from the airport. The powerful bonding process between us had already begun. Bitsy was taking in my face, my smells, my heartbeat, my voice. She was rapidly becoming very comfortable with me—something almost impossible to occur if she had been just a couple of weeks older.

When we arrived home from the airport, Peggy, Christie,

and Brian oohed and aahed for a little while as they stroked the tiny gray furball with the tips of their index fingers. Then the baby squirrel jumped from my shoulder to Peggy's, eventually settling down inside the pocket of Peggy's pajama top, this time with a pecan. Wow! This was even cozier than the last pocket!

"Oh, she's so itsy-bitsy!" Peggy whispered. And that's how Rocky's new gal pal ended up with the name Bitsy.

Bitsy has her own little cage next to Rocky's. They've gone nose to nose several times now and seem very interested in getting to know each other better. But let's be honest, Bitsy's seven weeks old and Rocky's seven years. She's too young!

In a few weeks, when she is a little bit bigger and more mature, we will start putting her in with Rocky for a few minutes at a time. By the end of thirty days or so, we hope she'll be blissfully living with the Rockster full-time.

Then, if we've truly helped create a marriage made in heaven, a year from now Rocky and Bitsy will be the proud parents of Rocky Two, Three, and maybe Four, along with a Rockette or two. Rocky seems excited by the whole prospect, especially when they touch noses, with Rocky trying to sneak kisses from her whenever we provide him the chance. This will be Rocky's first big opportunity to get a little tail, if you know what I mean.

The Rock even seems to be cutting back on his diet of pecans and walnuts. He appears to be eating more apples and oranges—more fresh fruit in general. I guess he wants to look as good as rodently possible when he's lying in the nesting box beside his young bride. Even though he's getting a little long in the tooth, Rocky still has his pride.

It's going to be a very fun next couple of years around here. If you want, I'll write another book about Rocky and Bitsy's adventures in paradise. I'll fill you in on their married life together and bring you up-to-date on what's happening up in the good old family tree. I'll give you the full report on their kids, including the good, the bad, and the ugly. But only if you want me to. Only if this book has entertained, inspired, and educated you, and warmed your heart and soul. Maybe even made you laugh out loud a time or two.

And if this book has succeeded in doing that for you, I'd love to hear about it. Just visit my web site or send me a letter:

Bill Goss and Rocky the Flying Squirrel
PO Box 7060
Orange Park, Florida 32073
USA

or

www.BillGoss.com

I'll try to get back to you as soon as I can. And if I can't, Rocky will. He's not flying around nearly as much as I am lately.

Acknowledgments

First, a tremendous thank you to my literary agent, Freya Manston. Without her unwavering faith in this project and in myself, without her initiative, vision, and drive, this book would simply not exist. Thank you to my editor, Brenda Copeland, and her predecessor, Tracy Bernstein, for skillfully slicing and dicing and yet keeping my voice intact. More important, they encouraged me to expand this book's scope beyond a cute little story about a Navy pilot and a flying squirrel. Instead, they asked that it encompass a whole lot more: health, cancer, the immune system, flying, the military, homeland defense, family, friends, faith—and the power of nature and the human spirit to supercharge our lives. And a special thanks to Judith Curr, publisher of Atria Books, for being touched by—and seeing the value of—this project the moment she heard about it.

Acknowledgments

There's a whole host of others I'd like to express my appreciation to, and so—especially if you're not mentioned in the body of this book somewhere else—I will try to do so now. Thank you to my great friends Dr. Marty Becker and James Bradley. Thank you to my wonderful lifelong friends Jeff Marcketta, Dave Graziano, Jim Mardis, Sandy North, Steve Kauffman, Bill Beck, Al Speidell, Frank Gren, and all of "The Men" whom I spent my boyhood with at "The Hotel" in Blairstown, New Jersey. And a special thanks to all their parents for tolerating us in their homes when we were truly intolerable.

Thank you to my fellow aviators in the United States military, particularly those in the U.S. Navy.

Thank you to Peggy, Christina, and Brian for giving me the greatest family and home a man could ever want. Thanks to all of my extremely tolerant siblings, to my in-laws, to my cousins, nieces, and nephews. Thanks to the many kind and generous people I've met in my studies and travels all over the globe, and to the wonderful medical professionals who have kept a watchful eye over me during some of my misadventures.

Other people—and their better halves—that I want to personally thank are Jimmy Angel, Billy Beal, Bruce Brownstein, Christine Clifford, Mike Delvecchio, Kelsea Eckart, Curtis Falgatter, Dave Faraldo, Doug Finnegan, Jamie Fee, Carolyn Herman, Jay Hanson, Glori Graziano, Mark Johnson, Denny Lott, Jason Maderski, Tom Marsland, Adam Merims, Don Milburn, Joe McCormick, Charlie Patton, Barbara Parker, Jack Prendergast, Larry Rayko, Zip Rausa, Bob Rippee, Bill Roelke, Larry Small, Lou Siracusano, Larry Smith, Milt Thomas, Bob Vito, Brian Washington, and Bill Yardley.

Now, if I've forgotten someone, well, I'm sorry, you know who you are . . . but please buy this book anyway.

Finally, I want to thank God for creating all the creatures—

no matter how great or small, no matter how scaly, toothy, slimy, feathered, or furred—that have slithered, crawled, climbed, hopped, or flown into my life and into my heart, blessing me with laughter and helping to save me from cancer.

Especially the littlest and liveliest angel you ever sent down here—Rocky the Flying Squirrel.